THE GREAT PHYSICIAN'S

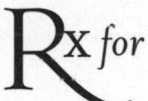 Rx *for*

IRRITABLE BOWEL SYNDROME

NELSON BOOKS
A Division of Thomas Nelson Publishers
Since 1798

www.thomasnelson.com

Published in Nashville, Tennessee, by Thomas Nelson, Inc.

Nelson Books titles may be purchased in bulk for educational, business, fundraising, or sales promotional use. For information, please e-mail SpecialMarkets@ThomasNelson.com.

Library of Congress Cataloging-in-Publication Data

Rubin, Jordan.
    The Great Physician's Rx for Irritable Bowel Syndrome / Jordan Rubin, with Joseph Brasco.
      p. cm.
    ISBN 0-7852-1416-X (hardcover)
    1. Irritable colon—Prevention—Popular works. 2. Irritable colon—diet therapy—Popular works. 3. Irritable colon—Religious Aspects—Christianity. I. Brasco, Joseph. II. Title.
RC862.R83 2006
616.3'42—dc22   2006013991

Printed in the United States of America

1 2 3 4 5 6 QW 09 08 07 06

CONTENTS

INTRODUCTION

An Embarrassing Health Problem

I've met some remarkable women over the years—including the love of my life, my wife, Nicki—but there's another Nicole who ranks right up there.

Nicole Yorkey was born in Basel, Switzerland, the eldest child of Hans and Thea Schmied. Her father was an engineer for one of the largest power-producing firms in Switzerland—an intelligent man who oversaw the construction of huge dam projects high in the Alps as well as Switzerland's first nuclear power plant. Her mother grew up in an apartment atop the family restaurant, where she and her six brothers and sisters were expected to pitch in from dawn until late at night: peeling potatoes in the kitchen, washing dishes and flatware, and waiting on customers.

Nicole's mother tongue was Swiss-German, a guttural language related to German but one that Germans in Berlin or Munich can't comprehend. Beginning in the first grade, Nicole and her classmates were taught the basics of "high" German, since this was the language used in Swiss newspapers, books, government offices, and official correspondence. The Swiss converse with each other in Swiss-German but write to each other in German. (I hope that's not too confusing.)

By the time Nicole reached high school, she was taking three more language classes: French, Italian, and English. In

Switzerland, the more languages you spoke, the better job you landed, and her parents encouraged her—even expected her—to do well in school. Her English teacher, however, wasn't encouraging at all, telling her on one occasion that she would never learn the language of the Anglo-Saxons. Still, she persevered, and her English improved when she traveled to London at age nineteen to live for six months with a family as an au pair.

Nicole's schoolbook Italian was very good, but her French was near perfect because the family owned a chalet in Villars, an Alpine ski resort town situated in the French-speaking part of Switzerland. Every weekend and winter holiday, she carved turns with her French-speaking friends from the time the lifts opened at nine in the morning to the last run at five o'clock. This Swiss Miss could really ski the bumps, and after she passed her Swiss certification test, she could teach anywhere in the world.

Armed with five different languages and her prized Swiss certification, Nicole turned her eyes toward America. Teaching a ski season in the States, she reasoned, would perfect her English and allow her to get an excellent job back in Switzerland. She wrote several dozen ski-school directors in the United States, including Max Good, who headed the ski school at Mammoth Mountain, a resort in California's Eastern Sierra. Max was also Swiss, and every year he brought over a half dozen Swiss ski instructors to round out his ski school and have instructors on hand who could teach European visitors in French, German, or Italian.

I'll let Nicole pick up her story here:

I met Mike Yorkey at the end of the season, just weeks before I was going to leave California and return home. As fate would have it, we fell in love and got married a year later.

This happened twenty-seven years ago, and since then, we've raised two children, Andrea and Patrick. I love cooking for the family, and I taught my children that enjoying food is an important part of Swiss culture. As for myself, I love eating various Swiss cheeses: Gruyere, Appenzeller, and Emmentaler, the latter being Switzerland's oldest and most important cheese because of its distinct nutty-sweet, mellow flavor. Emmentaler is the cheese with holes in it; here in the States, it's sold as "Swiss cheese." I also love mushrooms, mocha yogurts, cashews, and dried fruit.

The problem is that those foods don't like me. For years, I suffered terrible stomach pains whenever I ate these delicious items. Stress from tight finances or trying to do too many things at once were also enough to launch an attack on my digestive system. One time Mike had to run me to the emergency room because the abdominal pains felt like someone was stabbing me with a knife. Following another painful episode, I made an appointment with a gastroenterologist, who listened to my symptoms and ordered an upper and lower GI test for me. I didn't know what these English phrases meant, but I soon found out. For the lower GI, the doctor gave me so many drugs that the experience was bearable, but I can't say that having a nurse and doctor stick a tube with a camera into my backside was a pleasant incident.

When the results came back, I was told that there was nothing majorly wrong with me—no cancer, no polyps, no ulcerative colitis, and no Crohn's disease, but my colon was very spastic, meaning that it was constantly convulsive. "You have spastic colitis," said my doctor as he explained to me that spastic colitis was one of the handful of functional digestive disorders collectively known as irritable bowel syndrome or IBS. "You'll always have this because there is no cure for it," he said. My doctor then showed me a short video about IBS and mentioned that the best I could hope for was to listen to my stomach and stay away from foods that caused me pain. But how could I say no to dairy such as cheese and yogurt? I grew up with those simple foods and loved them. What else was I going to eat for breakfast or lunch? The doctor also gave me a prescription for a bottle of pills, but they made me feel so sick to my stomach that I never touched them again.

Then my husband, an author and editor who helps others write their books, was asked by Jordan Rubin to assist him with the writing and editing of *The Great Physician's Rx for Health and Wellness*. Jordan came to our house for planning sessions, and I helped out by transcribing their interviews.

What Jordan said about healthy living made sense to me, but I needed some practical help too. That's when Jordan told me he had developed a health plan based on the Bible and a dietary supplement with probiotics called soil-based organisms (SBOs) to help people like me with digestive problems. He offered me a sample bottle.

What a difference! I'd take my probiotic supplement, eat my Gruyere and Appenzeller cheese, and experience no pain! No longer did I have to cross my fingers when I diced mushrooms or reached for a mocha yogurt. Since then, I've been telling all my girlfriends about these supplements because a lot of them have the same abdominal issues that I do.

Nicole is being very gracious, and it's been great getting to know her and Mike. She invited Nicki and me to join them at the family chalet in Switzerland, and let me tell you: there's nothing better than traveling around Switzerland and Europe with someone who speaks five languages or enjoying a Swiss cheese fondue as you gaze at the snow-capped Alps.

Nicole loves dipping a wedge of old country bread into a fondue pot and enjoying a pain-free cheese fondue. She's grateful she can eat dairy products and simple Swiss foods without terrible abdominal cramps, dreadful bloating, and knifelike jabs in the gut—the classic symptoms of irritable bowel syndrome.

This will come across sounding like a cliché, but I know what Nicole has gone through. When I was nineteen—the same age as Nicole when she traveled to London to learn English—I worked as a summer camp counselor following my freshman year at Florida State University. I'll never forget the week I began experiencing nausea, stomach cramps, and horrible digestive problems out of the blue. The constant diarrhea was the worst. I'd be out on the ropes course with the kids when suddenly I'd have this gigantic urge to use the bathroom. After excusing myself to the other counselors, I'd walk *very quickly*—running was out of the question—to the nearest toilet, which was one of those hole-in-the-floor jobs. It was humiliating!

The relief never lasted long enough. An hour or two later, I'd have to make the same mad dash for the primitive toilets. My energy was sapped by the relentless diarrhea, causing me to lose twenty pounds in just six days. I became one sick puppy and had to leave camp.

That was the start of a two-year health odyssey that began with symptoms of IBS and developed into an inflammable bowel disease—Crohn's disease. (Irritable bowel syndrome is often mistaken for inflammatory bowel diseases like Crohn's disease or ulcerative colitis, but they're not the same.) I eventually reached a point where I thought I would have been better off dying because of the searing pain in my gut and around-the-clock diarrhea. I probably used the toilet one to two dozen times a day, and most of the time I was bleeding. Nighttime was the worst: I rarely slept more than forty-five minutes to an hour before I had to get to the bathroom

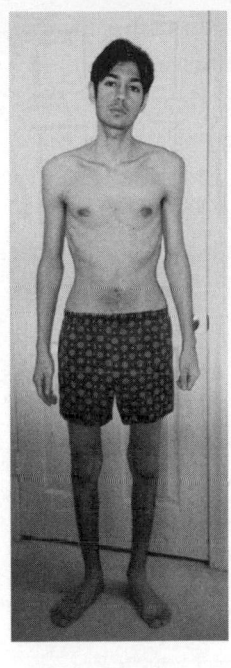

in a hurry. I shed pounds like a booster rocket roaring into space. At my lowest point, I wasn't much more than a stick figure, someone who weighed 104 pounds and resembled a Nazi death camp survivor.

I eventually made a full recovery by employing many of the principles that I share in *The Great Physician's Rx for Irritable Bowel Syndrome*. Today, at the age of thirty-one, God has blessed me with excellent health, and my painful digestive symptoms are in my rearview mirror. Although my digestive troubles were horrible, and I wish it upon no one, I also know that God didn't waste my painful experiences. I wrote about my health challenges—and, more importantly, provided solutions for many digestive problems—in a book I co-authored with Dr. Joseph Brasco called *Restoring Your Digestive Health*. (You'll learn more about this book in chapter one.)

The book's release prompted those with IBS and inflammatory bowel disease (IBD) to write or call me for advice. At speaking engagements, I can't tell you how many hurting folks pulled me aside to describe how their digestive issues made their lives miserable. Quite frankly, I learned more about other people's bowel habits than most would care to know, but that's been fine with me since I look at this as a ministry. Irritable bowel syndrome is a poorly understood disorder, but I've been there, and I understand it.

Since you're reading this book, I figure that you're dealing with a similar bowel disturbance or even excruciating abdominal pain. Or you're witnessing a family member deal with painful episodes of IBS. If so, please know that I'm writing *The Great Physician's Rx for Irritable Bowel Syndrome* for you and your loved one. I can't promise that either of you will be cured by the time you finish this book—this disorder has no known cure—but I can offer you an approach that will greatly increase your chances of living a normal life without intense abdominal pain.

AN AWKWARD SUBJECT

Irritable bowel syndrome is not a disease, but a painful, life-altering, functional digestive disorder in which the muscular contractions of the digestive tract become irregular and uncoordinated. IBS goes by other names as well: spastic colon, mucus colitis, spastic colitis, nervous stomach, or irritable colon. *The Encyclopedia of Natural Healing* says that in well over 80 percent of cases, tests reveal the presence of an overgrowth of fungi, parasites, or pathogenic bacteria. In addition, a change in the number and strength of intestinal contractions that push food through the intestine causes IBS. When the waves are faster and stronger, the contractions cause diarrhea; when the waves are slower, constipation follows.[1] Anxiety and emotional tension—those "butterflies in your stomach" or gut feelings—can adversely affect IBS symptoms and bring on an attack.

The very nature of IBS's symptoms—painful cramps, frequent flatulence, and alternating constipation and diarrhea—makes it difficult to discuss with family members, work colleagues, or friends. You don't see 10k walks, Labor Day telethons, or people pinning pink ribbons to their lapels (as they do for breast cancer awareness) or wearing canary yellow plastic wristbands (like those promoted by cyclist Lance Armstrong for cancer research) to create public awareness for IBS.

No one enjoys chatting about his or her personal bathroom habits—unless you're a stand-up comedian seeking a cheap laugh. I know that when I was a teenage camp counselor, I felt horrified when a buddy commented, "Hey, Jordan, how come you're running to the bathroom all the time? Is something wrong with you?" IBS is a closet disease, too embarrassing to bring up at the dinner table or discuss around the company watercooler. No wonder fewer than half of those enduring IBS symptoms seek medical attention.

Called "America's hidden health problem," IBS accounts for $25 billion in direct and indirect costs each year. Only the common cold causes more absenteeism in the workplace, according to Heather Van Vorous, author of *The First Year—IBS*.[2] Those who cope with this condition pay a heavy emotional cost for the pain and suffering visited upon them by this digestive affliction. You always have to know where the nearest bathroom is, since the urge to go can strike at any time. It's mentally draining always being on the lookout for a restroom. For those with IBS who travel a great deal, the phrase "Don't leave home without it" doesn't refer to their American Express card, but rather to their *Where to Stop and Where to Go* guide published by travel expert Arthur Frommer.

An estimated 30 million men, women, and children in this country—10 percent of the population—are plagued by persistent IBS symptoms, but many health experts believe that up to 20 percent of our population endure some form of bowel distress.[3] Maybe it's higher: a RoperASW national survey conducted in 2005 found that 43 percent of respondents suffered from recurring constipation, abdominal pain, or discomfort and bloating.[4] Chronic constipation brings on hemorrhoids, diverticulosis, and polyp formation.

IBS is an equal-opportunity condition that strikes both sexes at all ages, but the disorder falls heavily on women. Twice as many women are diagnosed with IBS as men, although some say that's because guys are more reluctant to see a doctor than women. Whether young or old, male or female, millions with IBS suffer in silence for two reasons: (1) they are unaware of the true impact of the disorder, and (2) they aren't sure what they can do to improve their condition.

Most people encountering irritable bowel syndrome note a dull pain in the lower abdomen or irregularity with their bowel movements. They will have recurrent diarrhea or constant constipation, or both in alternation. Sometimes their intestinal queasiness leads to bouts of flatulence. Since just about everyone has suffered from an occasional bowel disturbance at one time or another, most people learn to endure these discomforts. Unfortunately, an overwhelming 70 percent of those with IBS symptoms don't see a doctor. The remaining 30 percent experience enough pain and suffering that they can't put off seeing a doctor any longer. Even though so few—percentage wise—make it to a doctor's office, IBS is still the most common digestive disorder seen by physicians.

After making an appointment with their family doctor, many

find it embarrassing to discuss their bowel issues—or they wait until the doctor is halfway out the door before mentioning an embarrassing symptom. (For advice on this ticklish topic, log on to www.Take10forGIHealth.org and click on "Questions to ask.") Once the issue is on the table, physicians ask more questions. They conduct blood tests and sometimes order abdominal X-rays to make a diagnosis.

More often, however, family physicians refer you to an internal medicine specialist or gastroenterologist. As Nicole Yorkey learned, these specialists use the Rome II Diagnostic Criteria to properly diagnose irritable bowel syndrome. They are looking for at least two of the three following statements to be true:

1. Your painful symptoms are greatly relieved by a bowel movement.

2. There's been a change in the frequency of bowel movements.

3. There's been a change in the appearance (form) of the stool.

Nothing like getting down to the nitty-gritty, right? Doctors will also ask the following questions:

- Are you having bowel movements more than three times a day or less than three times a week?

- What does your stool look like? Lumpy and hard or loose and watery?

- Do you really have to strain to push a bowel movement out? After you go, do you feel like you could go again?

- Are you passing mucus in your stool?

- Do you feel bloated or have abdominal distension, which is the abnormal enlargement of the abdominal cavity caused by an accumulation of fluids and gas in the colon?

Doctors will also be interested in whether you've been experiencing fatigue, muscle pain, sleep disturbances, or sexual dysfunction. These symptoms may overlap or coexist with other conditions such as fibromyalgia, chronic fatigue syndrome, and interstitial cystitis.[5]

CONVENTIONAL TREATMENT

To the medical community, IBS is a "functional" disorder in which "the primary abnormality is an altered physiological function rather than an identifiable structural or biochemical cause," according to the International Foundation of Functional Gastrointestinal Disorders.

Translation: while medical researchers have yet to pinpoint an exact cause of IBS, they are confident that symptoms are produced by abnormal function of the nerves and muscles of the bowels. Something in the interaction between the gut, the brain, and the autonomic nervous system goes haywire, causing the bowel to become irritated and overly sensitive. Stress can be deadly.

I certainly believe that stress contributed to my intestinal problems. When I began college at Florida State University, I tried out for and made the Seminole cheerleading squad. Not bad for a freshman, but I was informed that if I missed one practice, I was off the squad. Did I mention that we practiced six days a week?

I also quarterbacked an intramural football team, served in church ministry, sang with a traveling church music group, and was chaplain of my fraternity. I was running from one thing to the next, hanging out with my friends, and studying into the wee hours. Stress was causing my digestive problems to bubble like a cauldron, ready to boil over at any moment.

Although some well-meaning friends may say that IBS "is in your mind," or that some type of psychological disorder brought on the symptoms, many in the medical community agree that stress can exacerbate or trigger symptoms. Physicians also feel they're on solid ground if they name your diet as the culprit.

When doctors make an IBS diagnosis, they usually suggest that you avoid problem foods such as dairy products and beans, as well as foods or drinks containing caffeine or fructose. They may have you work with a dietician to identify foods that aggravate your condition. Doctors will urge you to add high-fiber brown rice, oatmeal, barley, and vegetables to your meal plans.

If constipation is the culprit, physicians may suggest over-the-counter fiber supplements and laxatives containing bisacodyl (like Dulcolax), glycerin (like Fleet suppositories), and magnesium (like Milk of Magnesia) to soften stools and get things moving in the large intestine again. The value of laxatives for treating constipation-related IBS is a mixed bag since their efficacy is often unsatisfactory.

When stools are loose or diarrhea is unremitting, however, doctors may recommend an antidiarrheal like Loperamide, which slows the rate of food traveling through the stomach and intestines. The drug also acts to increase stool density and reduce the amount of fluid in the stool. Side effects, which are said not to be common, include difficulty breathing, swelling of the lips, tongue, or face, development of a fever, and persistent diarrhea.

In the last decade, giant pharmaceutical companies have poured hundreds of millions of research and development dollars into developing drugs that relieve IBS symptoms. So far, only two prescription drugs have been approved by the Food and Drug Administration for IBS: Lotronex and Zelnorm. Each has received mixed results.

The pharmaceutical company GlaxoSmithKline introduced Lotronex to considerable fanfare in early 2000, but the Food and Drug Administration yanked the drug off the market eight months later following the deaths of five women. (The drug doesn't work for men, but the FDA, which monitored testing, failed to state why.) Several dozen users also complained of severe constipation and ischemic colitis, which is the inflammation of the large bowel caused by reduced blood flow.

About 300,000 women were taking Lotronex under a doctor's supervision, and many felt helped. Thousands of women mailed letters of protest to the FDA, demanding the return of

Lotronex. The FDA relented in 2002 but tacked on restrictions limiting a doctor's ability to prescribe it. Sales have been far lower than expected, especially because GlaxoSmithKline declares that Lotronex poses serious risks and is only for women with severe diarrhea and IBS symptoms.

Zelnorm, manufactured by Novartis Pharmaceuticals of Switzerland, increases the action of serotonin (a hormone) in the intestines. This also-for-women-only drug speeds the movement of stools through the bowels. The main side effect, as you would expect for an anticonstipation drug, is diarrhea.

Zelnorm hasn't received widespread acceptance, and the International Foundation for Functional Gastrointestinal Disorders notes that no single medication on the U.S. market has been demonstrated in well-controlled clinical trials to be superior to a placebo for the treatment of IBS.

ALTERNATIVE TREATMENTS

Herbal medicine practitioners often use enteric-coated peppermint oil to treat IBS. Peppermint oil is said to inhibit gastrointestinal muscle contractions and excessive gas as well as soothe the touchy intestinal tract. Herbs such as chamomile, valerian, rosemary, and balm are promoted as having an antispasmodic effect on the intestines.[6]

Since many believe that IBS is a stress-related digestive problem, mind-body techniques such as biofeedback, yoga, hypnosis, and relaxation therapy are often employed. With biofeedback, a therapist shows you how to use an electronic monitor—known as a neuromuscular reeducation tool—to sense and control muscular activity in the digestive tract. By viewing a monitor that displays bodily functions, you receive information on how the body works so that you can retrain yourself to more normal functions.

Those who promote yoga for IBS say this mind-body therapy slows the respiratory rate, lowers blood pressure, and stabilizes digestion through exercise, breathing, and meditation, the latter being an anathema to Christians because of yoga's Eastern religion roots.

In hypnosis, a trained therapist teaches you the steps to enter a hypnotic state by focusing on breathing and imagining what it feels like to be relaxed and pain-free. Unlike the popular portrayal of hypnosis in films, on Jay Leno's *The Tonight Show*, and on stage shows, clinical hypnotherapists don't snap their fingers and put you under their spell. Instead, they make verbal suggestions that put you in a special mental state. Although proponents can't explain how hypnosis influences IBS in a beneficial way, they claim success rates ranging from 70 to 95 percent, based on controlled trials of hypnotherapy.[7]

Relaxation therapy is very similar to yoga, in which IBS sufferers are directed to tune out stress-inducing thoughts. Therapists will direct you to lie down and then flex and relax muscles, starting with your feet and working slowly toward your neck and shoulders.

Finally, another alternative treatment is applying Swedish bitters, a centuries old, dark brown, strong-smelling liquid containing a combination of herbs, to the hurting abdominal area and covering with a warm pack.

WHERE WE GO FROM HERE

I counsel a different approach to irritable bowel syndrome, which is based on the 7 Keys to unlocking your God-given health potential found in my foundational book, *The Great Physician's Rx for Health and Wellness*. These keys are the following:

- Key #1: Eat to Live
- Key #2: Supplement Your Diet with Whole Food Nutritionals, Living Nutrients, and Superfoods
- Key #3: Practice Advanced Hygiene
- Key #4: Condition Your Body with Exercise and Body Therapies
- Key #5: Reduce Toxins in Your Environment
- Key #6: Avoid Deadly Emotions
- Key #7: Live a Life of Prayer and Purpose

In the next seven chapters, I will show you how each of these keys directly or indirectly relates to IBS. I am convinced that adopting these 7 Keys will afford you an excellent chance to greatly reduce the intestinal distress that plagues you or a loved one. I believe each and every one of us has a God-given health potential that can be unlocked only with the right keys. I want to challenge you to incorporate these timeless principles and allow God to transform your health physically, mentally, emotionally, and spiritually.

KEY #1

Eat to Live

Let's say that thirty minutes after finishing a meal, a thumping headache bounces around the inside of your skull like a leaded Pachinko ball. Your stomach gurgles like Mount St. Helens, and you know what's coming next: a sprint to the nearest throne before the volcano explodes.

Eat.

Get diarrhea.

Eat.

Get diarrhea.

Eat.

Get diarrhea.

Spot a pattern here?

Eating is never any fun if you're sitting on porcelain half the day. In the midst of my digestive troubles during my college years, I dreaded every meal because I knew where I would eventually be heading. Sooner or later, though, I *had* to eat, so I lived on bland chicken soup, butternut squash, and pureed peas with the skin taken off. Gerber babies had it better than I did.

I tried dozens of diets, some mainstream, some faddish. For instance, I stopped eating meat for a while. Then I drank large amounts of cabbage juice. Another diet called for the consumption of Chinese and Peruvian herbs, Japanese kampo, olive leaf extract, and shark cartilage. I even attempted the ultra-clear detoxification/elimination diet. Talk about a colon cleanse!

Then I heard about the Specific Carbohydrate Diet (SCD), popularized by biochemist Elaine Gottschall, author of *Breaking the Vicious Cycle*. Without going into many details, the Specific Carbohydrate Diet banned many carbohydrate foods, fluid dairy products, grains and grain products, potatoes, yams, bean sprouts, and soybeans. I contacted Mrs. Gottschall, and for a couple of months, this kind lady and I conversed nearly every day as we tweaked the diet to cure my dreadful digestive problems. I stayed on the SCD diet for nearly six months with fanatical adherence, but it failed to reverse my condition, although thousands of others have said the Specific Carbohydrate Diet made a huge difference in calming their digestive tracts.

My battle with intestinal disorders lasted two years. During that time, I was bedridden with daily bouts of nausea, fever, night sweats, loss of appetite, severe abdominal cramps, and bloody diarrhea. I saw seventy doctors and medical practitioners (both traditional and alternative), including several gastroenterologists. They conducted a battery of tests, including the dreaded upper and lower GI and the unpleasant barium swallow.

The verdict: I had one of the worst cases of Crohn's disease they had ever come across. One of my doctors feared I would have to opt for the surgical removal of virtually all my large intestine and some of my small intestine. In surgical terms, doctors called it a colostomy. In practical terms, it meant I would have to wear bags attached to my abdominal wall to handle my bodily waste.

To a twenty-one-year-old on the cusp of adult life, that sounded like a death sentence. But I had no choice; I had run out of options. I was nothing more than skin and bones, a 104-pound skeleton close to death.

A week before my surgery, an acquaintance of my father called from San Diego. "I know why your son is not well," he began. "He's not following the health plan in the Bible."

Health plan in the Bible? I had read more than three hundred health books in the search for a cure, but not the Bible. I immediately grabbed my concordance and looked up every Scripture that had to do with health, food, and healing. What caught my attention was that God had given us a wonderful array of "natural" foods to eat, but our modern-day culture preferred inexpensive deep-fried, greasy foods high in calories, high in fat, high in sugar, and—in most people's minds—high in taste.

I started feasting on the Word of God and ate what God said to eat. I'll share specifics in a moment, but what I did can be boiled down to a pair of foundational thoughts that you can follow:

1. Eat what God created for food.
2. Eat food in a form that is healthy for the body.

I'm here to tell you that God healed my body in forty days. I gained twenty-nine pounds during that time, and while my healing wasn't instantaneous, it was miraculous nonetheless. To eat without pain and subsequent diarrhea felt like heaven on earth.

I want you—the person suffering from IBS—to experience that same type of miracle. I can't promise you that following

Key #1 of *The Great Physician's Rx for IBS* will chase away your abdominal stress, diarrhea, or constipation entirely, but I am confident that these principles give you the best shot at experiencing a vibrant life.

Besides, hasn't every other approach failed?

AN INTRODUCTION IS IN ORDER

It's time for me to introduce Dr. Joseph Brasco, a board-certified physician in internal medicine and gastroenterology and my co-author for this book. I met Dr. Brasco in 1999 at a seminar on clinical nutrition. I had been asked to speak about my digestive tract problems and what I did to get well; sitting in the front row that afternoon was Dr. Brasco.

After my talk, Dr. Brasco introduced himself to me. For a gastroenterologist, he seemed pretty cool: late thirties, dark curly hair, hip clothes, and a calm and dignified persona. He was friendly with a warm bedside manner.

As I recall, he thanked me for my transparency and wondered if we could have lunch together to discuss the topic further. I replied, "By all means," but I couldn't get over how a specialist in gastroenterology was seeking *my* opinions on how diet affected digestive diseases and irritable bowel syndrome. In 1999, I was a fresh-faced twenty-three-year-old studying naturopathic medicine, not a medical school graduate like him, but I had life experiences and triumph in an area of medicine where he didn't often come across successful outcomes.

Most of his patients, he said over our meal, came into his office feeling miserable. They didn't have a serious disease like cancer or inflammatory bowel disease—just a bad case of bloating, periods of passing gas, alternating constipation, and diarrhea. They felt that life dealt them a raw hand.

There wasn't much he could do in a ten-minute office visit, Dr. Brasco explained. He would listen to his patients describe the ailment, then he usually suggested a certain medication. That's what medical physicians like himself had been trained to do: make the diagnosis, fill out the prescription form, and send patients on their way.

Except that they kept returning to his examination room, complaining about the same symptoms and wanting more than a bottle of pills. That's when he would prescribe an anti-spasmodic or make arrangements for an upper or lower GI. When the patients returned complaining of *more* abdominal pain, he would order a CT scan. While good for his billing department, the patient (or the insurance company) would spend several thousand dollars on tests, but would be no closer to feeling better than on the first day he or she walked into his clinic.

Dr. Brasco had been fascinated by nutrition in med school, but his residency at a big city hospital was an eye-opener: the people walking into the emergency room lived in gritty neighborhoods dotted with fried-chicken drive-thrus, chili hamburger stands, tacquerias, waffle shops, and every fast-food purveyor in the country. His patient load lived on junk food—and paid a high price with their health.

He tried to explain basic nutrition to his ailing patients. *Stay away from fast food. Eat more vegetables. Snack on an apple a day.*

He had been influenced by *Enter the Zone,* authored by Barry Sears, which set forth the idea that restricting carbohydrates may reduce bloating and other gastrointestinal problems for those with IBS. Dr. Brasco became an evangelist for the low-carbohydrate gospel with his patients. I wouldn't say that he got in their faces, but he was rather direct.

"Listen," he would say to his patients after hearing a litany of symptoms, "I'm convinced that you have irritable bowel syndrome. We have two ways of looking at this. I can prescribe a medicine for you, which will help a little bit, but you're going to be right back in this examination room one month from now complaining that your stomach hurts. Or, if you're interested, we can change your diet, but you will have to work with me. I don't want to waste my time or yours if you're not interested in making a major lifestyle change in what you choose to eat."

Dr. Brasco said that only a third of his patients were willing to say good-bye to deep-fried crispy chicken and hush puppies. The rest preferred to take their prescription in hand and wash down pills with water, even though prescription drugs—everything from Amitriptyline to Zantac—rarely calmed things down in the digestive tract. They weren't willing to make the hard choices that a lifestyle change involves.

Dr. Brasco knew what hard choices entailed since he had digestive issues of his own. He practiced what he preached, though, by shopping at health food stores and eating a diet heavy in whole grains while eschewing meat. He believed that a high-fiber diet—bananas, oatmeal, bran cereal—would make him feel better. A funny thing happened, however: the physician wasn't able to heal himself.

So Dr. Brasco continued his search, and that's the main reason he took me aside after I spoke at the seminar on clinical nutrition. He was eager to learn more about the diet that eventually healed me of my painful digestive ailments—a diet that's part of the Great Physician's prescription for health and wellness.

Are you willing to make big changes in what you eat? I believe you'll have to, but I see nothing but upside. Aren't you enormously interested in eating without experiencing excruciating pain? Haven't there been times when you said you'd do *anything* to feel better? Well, your chance has come. Dr. Brasco and I are in agreement that the most important thing you can do is make changes in your eating habits, because a poor diet plays a huge role with IBS.

What you're about to read in this chapter are principles for eating that have been adopted by both Dr. Brasco and myself to ease our own digestive problems. A book that we coauthored earlier together, *Restoring Your Digestive Health*, laid the foundation for the 7 Keys and *The Great Physician's Rx for Irritable Bowel Syndrome*. If you stick with us, you'll learn why Key #1, "Eat to Live," may be your best weapon against the scourges of irritable bowel syndrome.

MAKING A LIST AND CHECKING IT TWICE

When it comes to eating (1) foods that God created and (2) in a form healthy for the body, God declared in Genesis that He was giving Adam and Eve every seed-bearing plant and every tree with fruit for food (1:29) and plants of the field (3:18). In Deuteronomy, God presented the animals that people could eat: the ox, the sheep, the goat, the deer, the gazelle, the roe deer, the wild goat, the ibex, the antelope, and the mountain sheep. Elsewhere in Scripture God's people ate foods such as almonds, barley, beans, bread, cakes, cheese, cucumbers, onions, leeks, melons, curds of cow's milk, figs, fish fowl, fruit, game, goat's milk, grain, grapes, grasshoppers, herbs, honey, lentils, meal, pistachio nuts, oil, olives, quail, raisins, sheep, veal, and vegetables.

These foods I just listed are nutritional gold mines and contain no refined or processed carbohydrates and no artificial sweeteners. I'm convinced that a diet based on consuming whole and natural foods fits within the bull's-eye of "eating to live" and gives you the best chance to overcome IBS. Yet too many of the so-called foods sold in our nation's supermarkets are not created by God but are produced by employees in hairnets on an assembly line at some far-flung factory. Like sheep following the next one off a cliff, we fill our shopping carts with processed foods that do a number on our stomachs and provoke diarrhea and constipation problems. Processed foods strain the gut because the digestive tract must toil harder to extract nutrients from foods whose nutritional ingredients were raided before and during the manufacturing process.

But Jordan, if you're telling me to eat a bunch of natural foods for my IBS, it can't be this simple.

You're right. It's not that simple. You must consume your foods carefully, especially carbohydrates, which play a big part in IBS flare-ups. Every bite you take, whether it's a protein, fat, or carbohydrate, impacts your digestion—and therefore your symptoms. Let's take a closer look at these macronutrients.

PROTEINS ARE PRACTICALLY PERFECT

Proteins, one of the basic components of nutrition, are the essential building blocks of the body. All proteins are combinations of twenty-two amino acids, which build body organs, muscles, and nerves, to name a few important duties. Among other things, proteins provide for the transport of nutrients, oxygen, and waste throughout the body and are required for the structure, function, and regulation of the body's cells, tissues, and organs.

Our bodies, however, cannot produce all twenty-two amino acids that we need to live a robust life. Scientists have discovered that eight essential amino acids are missing, meaning that they must come from other sources outside the body. Since we need those eight amino acids badly, it just so happens that animal protein—chicken, beef, lamb, dairy, eggs, etc.— is the only complete protein source providing the Big Eight amino acids.

That's why vegetarianism, which Dr. Brasco and I tried in our desperation to feel better, was doomed for failure.

LOW FAT EQUALS LOW HEALTH

Before we began collaborating on *Restoring Your Digestive Health*, Dr. Brasco urged his patients to switch to low-fat foods, which are part of the mantra for by-the-medical-book advice: increase fiber and embrace a low-fat diet.

The problem with reduced-fat chips and fat-free cookies is more than their poor taste: chemically altered foods make things worse for the body, not better. Ron Rosedale, M.D., author of *The Rosedale Diet*, pointed out that laboratory animals, which live traumatic lives inside small cages, suffer from stress disorders and premature death. Yet, when these laboratory animals were fed a high-fat diet, the life-shortening effects of stress were alleviated. "The same appears to be true for humans," Dr. Rosedale writes. "Eating a low-fat diet can promote depression and anxiety in humans."[1] And we all know that stress and anxiety are not an IBS sufferer's best friend.

What type of fats in foods should those with IBS eat? The fat found in grass-fed animals, lamb, dairy products from grain-fed animals, wild-caught fish, free-range poultry, nuts, seeds, and nut and seed butters are great sources of fats. People are often shocked to hear me say this, but this is why I say butter is healthier for you than margarine. Butter, when organically produced, is loaded with healthy fatty acids such as short-chain saturated fatty acids, which supply energy to the body and aid in the regeneration of the digestive tract. Margarine, on the other hand, is a man-made, congealed conglomeration of chemicals and hydrogenated liquid vegetable oils.

Fats and oils created by God, as you would expect, are fats you want to include in your diet. The top two on my list are extra virgin coconut and olive oils, which are beneficial to the body and aid metabolism. I urge you to cook with extra virgin coconut oil, which is a near-miracle food that few people have ever heard of.

THE TRUTH ABOUT CARBOHYDRATES

Now comes the moment of truth about carbohydrates: those with IBS should restrict the consumption of carbohydrates and wisely choose the carbs they eat. One of the benefits of reducing carbohydrates is an improvement in intestinal flora, or bacterial microorganisms. Few people have heard of intestinal flora or are aware that there are trillions of cells in the human body but even more microbial cells in the large intestine in the form of intestinal flora. The body permits these friendly bacteria and yeasts to live in the intestinal tract because they are the first line of defense against disease-causing bacteria, viruses, toxins, and parasites.

By definition, carbohydrates are the sugars and starches contained in plant foods. Sugars and starches, like fats, are not bad for you, but the problem is that the standard American diet is weighted way too heavily on sugar-laden foods that come with every meal: breakfast with its sweet cereals, break time with soda or coffee mixed with sugar, lunch with its cookies, and dinner with its sugary desserts.

Sugar is known as a disaccharide sugar. Refined white sugar has a way of feeding the "bad" microorganisms in the intestines. One such organism, a yeast called *Candida albicans*, absolutely *loves* sugar. Eating too many sugary foods causes Candida and thrush to thrive and feeds harmful bacteria that irritate the lining of the GI tract.

Starches such as bread, pasta, rice, corn, and potatoes are disaccharide carbohydrates as well, which are more difficult to digest. The digestive system finds these type of carbohydrates to be the most difficult to break down. What happens in the digestive process is that some undigested carbohydrates remain in the small intestine instead of traveling on to the large intestine, where they can be eliminated from the body. When unabsorbed carbohydrates camp out in the small intestine, they feed harmful bacteria and upset the balance of the intestinal flora—a perfect storm for IBS to rear its ugly head.

The result—gas and acids caused by bacterial fermentation—becomes a vicious cycle, which is why Elaine Gottschall named her book *Breaking the Vicious Cycle*. Undigested carbohydrates encourage bacterial fermentation, and bacterial fermentation makes it more difficult for carbohydrates to be absorbed. As you continue eating disaccharide-rich foods, your body never has a chance to catch up.

In *The Great Physician's Rx for Irritable Bowel Syndrome*, I recommend that you avoid eating unnecessary sugar and cut back on your starches considerably. Avoiding sugar and its sweet relatives—high fructose corn syrup, sucrose, molasses, and maple syrup—is easier said than done.

The carbohydrates you want to consume are low glycemic, high nutrient, and low sugar. These would be most high-fiber fruits, especially berries, vegetables, nuts, seeds, and some legumes, plus a small amount of whole grain products (sprouted, soaked, or sour-leavened), which are always better than refined carbohydrates that have been stripped of their vital fiber, vitamin, and mineral components.

Eating unrefined carbohydrate foods introduces fiber-rich foods into your body. Fiber is the indigestible remnants of plant cells found in vegetables, fruits, whole grains, nuts, seeds, and beans. Fiber-rich foods take longer to break down and are partially indigestible, which means that as these foods work their way through the digestive tract, they absorb water and increase the elimination of fecal waste in the large intestine.

Good sources of fiber are berries, fruits with edible skins (apples, pears, and grapes), citrus fruits, whole non-gluten grains (quinoa, millet, amaranth, and buckwheat), green peas, carrots, cucumbers, zucchini, and tomatoes. Green leafy vegetables such as spinach are also rich in fiber. Eating foods high in fiber and low in starches will immediately improve your digestion as you begin to "starve off" the harmful microorganisms in your body.

Chewing your food well will greatly improve the digestion of carbohydrates. If people tease you about "inhaling" your food, then you're eating too fast. I recommend chewing each mouthful of food twenty-five to seventy-five times before swallowing. This advice may sound ridiculous, but I know that a conscious effort to chew food slowly ensures that plenty of digestive juices are added to the food as it begins to wind through the digestive tract. I can't emphasize enough the critical importance of chewing your food well when you have IBS.

THE GREAT PHYSICIAN'S NUTRITIONAL RECOMMENDATIONS

Now it's time to get to the nitty-gritty: What can you, as an IBS sufferer, eat? Let's go down the following list:

1. Meats.

I advocate eating organically raised cattle, sheep, goats, buffalo, and venison that graze on nature's bountiful grasses and fish caught in the wild like salmon, tuna, or sea bass. Grass-fed meat is leaner and is lower in calories than grain-fed beef. Organic and grass-fed beef is higher in gut-friendly omega-3 fatty acids and important vitamins like B_{12} and vitamin E, and way better for you than assembly-line cuts of flank steak from hormone-injected cattle eating pesticide-sprayed feed laced with antibiotics.

Fish with fins and scales caught from oceans and rivers are lean sources of protein and provide essential amino acids in abundance. Supermarkets are stocking these types of foods in greater quantities these days, and of course they are found in natural food stores, fish markets, and specialty stores.

You must avoid certain meats. I'm talking about breakfast links, bacon, lunch meats, ham, hot dogs, bratwurst, and other sausages. I have other reasons for recommending that you stay away from meats like bacon and ham lunch meat. In all of my previous books, I've consistently pointed out that pork—America's "other white meat"—should be avoided because pigs were called "unclean" in Leviticus and Exodus. God created pigs as scavengers—animals that survive just fine on any farm slop or water swill tossed their way. Pigs have a simple stomach arrangement: whatever a pig eats goes down the hatch, straight into the stomach, and out the back door in four hours max. They'll even eat their own excrement, if hungry enough.

Even if you decide to keep eating commercial beef instead of the organic version, I absolutely urge you to stop eating pork.

Read Leviticus 11 and Deuteronomy 14 to learn what God said about eating clean versus unclean animals, where Hebrew words used to describe "unclean meats" can be translated as "foul" and "putrid," the same terms that describe human waste.

Please realize that not all sea life is healthy to eat. Shellfish and fish without fins and scales, such as catfish, shark, and eel, are also described in Leviticus 11 and Deuteronomy 14 as "unclean meats." God called hard-shelled crustaceans such as lobster, crabs, shrimp, and clams unclean because they are "bottom feeders," content to sustain themselves on excrement from other fish. To be sure, this purifies water but does nothing for the health of their flesh.

Eating unclean foods fouls the body and may lead to IBS symptoms. God declared these meats unclean because He understands the ramifications of eating them, and you should as well.

2. Cultured dairy products from goats, cows, and sheep.

When I began following the diet of the Bible, I started consuming cultured dairy products such as yogurt and kefir from goat's and cow's milk. One benefit of eating cultured dairy is the beneficial microorganisms they contain. These living organisms contain something called "probiotics," which, by definition, are living, direct-fed microbials (DFMs) that promote the growth of beneficial bacteria in the intestines. The normal human gastrointestinal tract contains hundreds of different species of harmless or even friendly bacteria, otherwise known as intestinal flora, but when an unbalance of these bacteria occurs, the result is often constipation or diarrhea.

One of the best ways to introduce probiotics to your diet is through cultured dairy products such as raw goat's milk in the form of fermented kefir. Dairy products derived from goat's milk and sheep's milk can be easier on stomachs than those from cows, although dairy products from organic or grass-fed cows can be excellent as well. Goat's milk is less allergenic because it does not contain the same complex proteins found in cow's milk.

If you have IBS or other digestive problems, I recommend you avoid consuming fluid dairy products, such as milk and ice cream, since they contain the milk sugar lactose. Instead, I recommend eating fermented dairy products such as yogurt, kefir, hard cheeses, cultured cream cheese, cottage cheese, and cultured cream. Those who are lactose-intolerant—and many with IBS are sensitive to lactose—can often stomach fermented dairy products because they contain little or no residual lactose, which is the type of sugar in milk that many find hard to digest.

3. Cultured and fermented vegetables.

Raw cultured or fermented vegetables such as sauerkraut, pickled carrots, beets, or cucumbers supply the body with probiotics as well. Although these fermented vegetables are often greeted with upturned noses at the dinner table, these foods help reestablish natural balance to our digestive system. Cultured vegetables like sauerkraut are brimming with vitamins, such as vitamin C, and contain almost four times the nutrients as unfermented cabbage. The lactobacilli in fermented vegetables contain digestive enzymes that help break down food and increase its digestibility. I urge you to sample sauerkraut or pickled beets which are readily available in health food stores.

4. Fruits.

The Great Physician's Rx for Irritable Bowel Syndrome calls for the judicious intake of raw fruit, which is quite healthy but may cause digestive disturbances for those with IBS. If you're still having diarrhea problems, eat fruit cautiously. Because of its high sugar content, I do not recommend that you eat fruit on its own; fruit should be consumed with fats and proteins, which will slow down the absorption of sugar.

Limit your consumption to two or three fresh fruits daily, which can be consumed during snack time. For IBS health, I recommend blueberries, strawberries, raspberries, and grapes, fully ripened and organic. When it comes to keeping your stomach calm, I believe you should eat organic fruits and vegetables that have not been grown with pesticides or chemical fertilizers. Try to eat fruits and vegetables in season; no one enjoys eating rubbery half-green tomatoes. I'm fine with using frozen produce since that often represents the best option for healthy fruits and veggies in January. In the case of berries and certain fruits, the difference between fresh and frozen is minimal.

5. Spices.

A household spice in your cupboard may have IBS-reducing properties. Ginger, the world's most widely cultivated spice, contains chemicals that inhibit toxic bacteria in the digestive tract while it promotes friendly bacteria, which is why this spice is effective in treating conditions ranging from constipation to diarrhea. Ginger reduces the total volume of gastric juices, says Paul Schulick, author of *Ginger: Common Spice & Wonder Drug*. "From all parts of the world, virtually every ethnomedical text citing ginger has lauded its wide range of benefits to the digestive system," he writes.[2]

There's another spice, albeit rarely used, that aids in healing for those with IBS: peppermint. As I mentioned in the Introduction, peppermint oil taken in enteric-coated capsule form—which prevents the peppermint oil from being released until it reaches the colon—provides effective treatment for many irritable bowel symptoms. "Peppermint oil inhibits gastrointestinal smooth-muscle contraction and excessive gas," says the *Encyclopedia of Natural Healing*. "Peppermint oil provides effective treatment for many of the symptoms of an irritable bowel that is not complicated by infection."[5]

6. Water.

Water isn't a food, of course, but this calorie-free and sugar-free substance performs many vital tasks when it comes to digestion. First of all, the intestinal tract uses a lot of water to break down solid foods. Water acts as a lubricant to move things through the large intestine and assists in the solidifying and forming of stools. A healthy stool is made of water, undigested fiber, and living and dead bacteria. A stool that stays too long in the large intestine can dry out and be difficult to push out of the colon; this is known as constipation.

F. Batmanghelidj, M.D., author of *You're Not Sick, You're*

Thirsty!, said that water is the main solvent for all foods, vitamins, and minerals. Water breaks down food into smaller particles and their eventual metabolism and assimilation. "Water energizes food, and food particles are then able to supply the body with this energy during digestion," he writes. "This is why food without water has absolutely no energy value for the body."[4]

When it comes to digestive health, the best way to prevent constipation is to drink plenty of water—the proverbial eight glasses a day. Any less, and you're asking for abdominal trouble. In a healthy digestive tract, the body processes food from the time it enters the mouth until it's expelled in a twelve-to-twenty-four hour window. Food staying any longer than twenty-four hours pollutes the large intestine and contributes to constipation, so you need water to keep things moist, in motion, and moving along.

By contrast, diarrhea is a stool that contains too much water. So can you get diarrhea from drinking *too* much H_2O? No, diarrhea is not caused by swigging bottle after bottle of Aquafina; in fact, diarrhea is very dehydrating and steals water from the body. So you need to drink a lot of water even if you're battling a bad case of the runs.

You should drink a minimum of eight glasses of water a day to stay hydrated. Sure, you'll need to urinate more often, which means even *more* visits to the bathroom, but is that so bad? Drinking plenty of water is not only healthy for the body, but it's a key part of the Great Physician's Rx for IBS Battle Plan (see page 72), so keep a water bottle close by and drink water before and during meals. Do most of your water drinking between meals, and stay away from ice-cold beverages. Ice-cold drinks shock the system and temporarily shut down digestion, not a good development for someone fighting IBS.

This seems like a good place to talk about this country's obsession with coffee, thanks to your neighborhood Starbucks. For those with IBS, I would urge you to stay away from coffee. This substance is too taxing on the esophagus and digestive tract, and caffeine stresses out the adrenal glands and makes the body more susceptible to disease and infection.

Teas and herbal infusions (the latter beverage is made from herbs and spices, rather than the actual tea plant) are a better story all together. My favorite tea blends contain combinations of tea (green, black, or white) with biblical herbs and spices such as grape, pomegranate, hyssop, olive, and fig leaves. Even though I've never thought of myself as a tea-drinking type, my wife, Nicki, and I enjoy these biblical tea blends with meals.

You'll find in my Great Physician's Rx for IBS Battle Plan (see page 72) that I recommend a cup of hot tea and honey with breakfast, dinner, and snacks. I also advise consuming freshly made iced tea, as tea can be consumed hot or steeped and iced. Please note that while herbal tea provides many great health benefits, nothing can replace pure water for hydration. Although you can safely and healthfully consume two to four cups of tea and herbal infusions per day, you still need to drink at least eight cups of pure water for all the good reasons I've described in this section.

Practice Fasting Once a Week

If your stomach does a break-dance every time you eat a sandwich or your gut spasms in pain following a meat-and-potatoes dinner, then I urge you to practice a partial fast once a week. I'm a firm believer in the value of giving the body's midsection time off from the round-the-clock digestive cycle, which could ease abdominal stress and pains. The pancreas gets a rest because it doesn't have to produce the digestive enzymes needed to process foods.

For those with IBS, I think it's better—and more realistic—to concentrate on completing a one-day partial fast once a week. In this type of fast, you wake up in the morning and refrain from eating breakfast and lunch, as well as any snacks. Then you resume eating with a dinnertime meal.

Fasting is a form of discipline that isn't easy for someone who's never done it. If you've never voluntarily fasted for a day, I urge you to try it—preferably toward the end of the week. I've found that Thursdays or Fridays work best for me because the week is winding down, and the weekend is coming up. For instance, I won't eat breakfast and lunch so that when I break my fast and eat dinner that night, my body has gone between eighteen and twenty hours without food or sustenance since I last ate dinner the night before.

If I had IBS, my attitude about fasting would be *What do I have to lose?* You may find that fasting is the pause that refreshes. Taking a sustained break from eating will improve your physical health in ways you can't understand, but there's a spiritual side to fasting that must be addressed as well. When you fast and pray (two words that seem to go hand in hand in Scripture), you are pursuing God in your life and opening yourself to experiencing a renewed sense of well being and dependence upon the Lord.

THE DIRTY DOZEN

Whether you're trying to avoid IBS outbreaks or you have someone in the family who has a sensitive stomach, here is a list of foods that should never find a way onto your plate or into your hands. I call them "The Dirty Dozen." Some I've already discussed elsewhere in this chapter, while the rest are presented here with a short commentary:

1. **Pork products.** These meats top my list because they are staples in the standard American diet and extremely unhealthy.

2. **Shellfish and fish without fins and scales, such as catfish, shark, and eel.** God also called hard-shelled crustaceans such as lobsters, crabs, and clams unclean in the Old Testament. Their flesh harbors known toxins that can contribute to poor health and set your digestive tract on edge. Am I saying *au revoir, sayonara,* and *adios* to lobster thermidor, shrimp tempura, and carnitas burritos? That's what I'm saying.

3. **Hydrogenated oils.** This means margarine and shortening are taboo, as well as any commercial cakes, pastries, desserts, and anything with the words "hydrogenated" or "partially hydrogenated" on the label.

4. Artificial sweeteners. Aspartame (found in NutraSweet and Equal), saccharine (Sweet 'N Low), and sucralose (Splenda) are chemicals several hundred times sweeter than sugar and found in every sit-down restaurant in America. More than 180 million Americans regularly reach for a packet. Do they cause stomach problems?

Sugar alcohols and polyols such as sorbitol, malitol, isomalt, and a whole lot of other scientific-sounding names are found in popular artificial sweeteners. Yes, Virginia, they can create GI problems. Dr. Prabhakar Swaroop, assistant professor of gastroenterology at Saint Louis University, says, "These sugar alcohols are made up of long chains, and our bodies have a hard time breaking them down." In large amounts, they can cause diarrhea, gas, and bloating—what people refer to as a "laxative effect," he adds.[5]

5. White flour. White flour isn't a problematic chemical like artificial sweeteners, but it's virtually worthless and not healthy for you.

6. White sugar. If you're looking for another culprit to blame, then jump on the sugar bandwagon.

7. Soft drinks. Run, don't hide, from this liquefied sugar. A twelve-ounce Coke or Pepsi is the equivalent of eating nearly nine teaspoons of sugar. Popular soft drinks also contain chemicals that cause the body to become more acidic, which is not a great feeling for the stomach.

8. Pasteurized homogenized skimmed milk. Like I said, whole organic milk is better, and goat's milk is even better; and if you have IBS, cultured or fermented dairy is the best.

9. Corn syrup. It's just another version of sugar but even more fattening.

10. Hydrolyzed soy protein. If you're wondering what in the world this is, hydrolyzed soy protein is found in imitation meat products. Stick to the real stuff.

11. Artificial flavors and colors. These are never good for you under the best of circumstances, and certainly not when you're trying to ease digestive pain.

12. Excessive alcohol. Although studies point out the benefits of drinking small amounts of red wine for the heart (known as the "French Paradox"), the fact remains that alcohol contains lots of sugars and calories. And overconsumption of alcohol has wrecked millions of families over the years.

EAT: WHAT FOODS ARE EXTRAORDINARY, AVERAGE, OR TROUBLE?

I've prepared a comprehensive list of foods that are ranked in descending order based on their health-giving qualities. Foods at the top of the list are healthier than those at the bottom. The best foods to serve and eat are what I call "Extraordinary," which God created for us to eat and will give you the best chance to live a long and happy life. If you have irritable bowel issues, it's best if at least 75 percent of your diet is made up of foods from the Extraordinary category.

Foods in the Average category should make up less than 50 percent of your daily diet. If you're struggling with IBS, it's best to limit consumption of Average foods to less than 25 percent of your daily diet.

Foods in the Trouble category should be consumed with extreme caution. If you're having an IBS flare-up, you should avoid these foods completely.

For the listing of Extraordinary, Average, and Trouble Foods, visit www.BiblicalHealthInstitute.com and click on "What to E.A.T.".

℞ THE GREAT PHYSICIAN'S RX FOR IBS: EAT TO LIVE

- *Eat only foods God created.*

- *Eat foods in a form healthy for the body.*

- *Try eating smaller meals throughout the day rather than three large ones.*

- *At mealtime consume protein, fat, and veggies before starchy carbohydrates.*

- *Restrict or avoid disaccharide-containing foods such as fluid dairy, unsprouted grains, sugar, corn, and potatoes.*

- *Drink at least eight or more glasses of pure water per day to properly hydrate your digestive tract.*

- *Partially fast one day per week to give your digestive system a break.*

- *Chew each mouthful of food twenty-five to seventy-five times.*

Take Action

To learn how to incorporate the principles of eating to live into your daily life, please turn to page 72 for the Great Physician's Rx for IBS Battle Plan.

KEY #2

Supplement Your Diet with Whole Food Nutritionals, Living Nutrients, and Superfoods

In the spring of 1997, I received a phone call from Dr. Morton Walker, a medical researcher and columnist for *Townsend Letter for Doctors & Patients*, a newsletter that publishes information about the latest news in alternative medicine written by researchers, health practitioners, and patients. Dr. Walker had been tipped off about the story of a twenty-one-year-old college student with Crohn's disease who regained his health by following a biblically based health plan and supplementing his diet with probiotics with soil-based organisms (SBOs).

That person would be me.

Dr. Walker and I had a friendly chat, and he wrote a lengthy article about my battle back from "death's door." The complimentary story was an exhaustive, detailed account of my chronic bowel abnormalities and two-year chase to find *something* that would allow me to resume a normal life.

That something turned out to be a four-thousand-year-old health plan that included the consumption of friendly microorganisms found in healthy plants and soil—living microbials that increased my ability to absorb nutrients from food while promoting the growth of beneficial bacteria in the intestines. I first learned of them while I was living for a short time in San Diego, where I was seeking an answer for my digestive ailments.

While in San Diego, my father, Dr. Herb Rubin, mailed an interesting looking package to me. Keep in mind that my father was a chiropractic doctor and naturopath who advocated holistic health and never allowed processed foods or anything with refined sugar to be brought into the home. He loved doing this sort of stuff. I opened Dad's package, only to find a plastic bag containing black-colored powder. A note had been attached: "I know I promised not to send you anything more to try, but I really think you should add this to your diet. Love, Dad."

Yeah, right. Had Dad already forgotten that I had tried and tested every supplement known to man, including thirty different probiotics? None of these supplements did anything special for me, although I could remember a couple of products that made me violently ill or touched off another round of diarrhea. Now my father was urging me to sample the substance in the plastic bag—a substance that sure looked like *dirt.*

I called my father in Florida to ask him what was up. After we exchanged pleasantries, he remained confident that the black powder was just the nature-based elixir I needed. "It may look like dirt, but it isn't," he promised. "That plastic bag contains healthy organisms and minerals from the soil." An article accompanying the package explained that nutrients had been hijacked from our soil-depleted farmlands. Not only were nutrients and trace minerals AWOL, the note said, but "living organisms" in our foods had been wiped out by three things: the pesticide treatment of cropland, pasteurization of dairy products, and modern man's disdain for microorganisms. As I peered into Dad's plastic bag of black powder, I thought, *What do I have to lose?*

Over the next week, I mixed some of this black powder in water and drank the dark-colored cocktail. It wasn't as bad as Rocky drinking raw eggs before a workout, but it wasn't much better. I had already decided to increase the amount of gut-friendly foods in my diet by seeking out foods containing these beneficial microorganisms: raw goat's or cow's milk in the form of fermented kefir, sprouts, organic fruits and vegetables, raw sauerkraut, and carrot and other vegetable juices.

These "live" foods, I had learned, retained their beneficial enzymes and microorganisms. The reason I tell you this is that after my health improved and I resumed a normal life, I continued to consume supplements made with soil-based organisms and other probiotic microorganisms, which are known in the natural health industry as "whole food" or "living" supplements or multivitamins.

I described everything I just told you to Dr. Walker, and he skillfully reconstructed my road back to health in an article that created quite a stir in the natural health industry. "The SBOs detoxified Jordan's intestinal tract, which reversed the degenerative process of his Crohn's disease," he writes, adding that I had been healed from this devastating illness.[1]

I don't know how many people read *Townsend Letter*, but I'm not exaggerating when I say that several thousand people contacted me asking about the diet and SBOs that helped me. Many of these letters and phone calls were from hurting folks with IBS and IBD symptoms who wanted to know where and how they could purchase this probiotic "dirt" supplement.

PROBIOTICS FOR IBS

I was only twenty-two years old, but I had a passion to transform people's health. I really thought I could help these people, and Lord knows I was touched by their descriptions of abdominal anguish. Necessity being the mother of invention, I set out to formulate my own probiotic supplement with SBOs. I did two things: I contacted the manufacturer of the SBO product I was using, then I searched all the available literature on probiotics and SBOs to see if any micronutrients could or should be added to the equation. Remember, I was earning my naturopathic degree at this time, so I was learning about the appropriate microorganisms that should be included in my formulation. I included several different beneficial microbes, including various Lactobacilli, Bacilli, and Sacchromyces species.

Nearly ten years laster, I still consume a probiotic supplement every day. In fact, hundreds of thousands of people have consumed the probiotic product I have formulated, and many have reported great results.

I'm telling this story not to puff myself up because what happened is clearly a God thing, but to show you that supplementing your diet with a probiotic containing SBOs can be an IBS sufferer's best friend (for recommended brands, visit www.BiblicalHealth Institute.com and click on the GPRx Resource Guide). I'm convinced, more than ever, that nutrients produced by probiotic fermentation—a process in which beneficial bacteria and yeasts are created into beneficial compounds—enhance digestive health.

That's why I urge you to supplement your diet with probiotics, whole food nutritionals, living nutrients, and superfoods.

STARTING WITH A GOOD MULTIVITAMIN

When I was a student of naturopathic medicine, I studied the work of Dr. Weston Price, a Cleveland dentist who lived from 1870 to 1948. As he filled more and more cavities of patients sitting in his dental chair, he wondered, *Could it be our processed foods causing these cavities?* Dr. Price left his practice and traveled around the world studying indigenous people whose teeth and gums were untouched by processed foods. He came into contact with fourteen primitive cultures who not only displayed row after row of healthy teeth, but these smiling men, women, and children also lived healthy lives virtually free of physical disease.

I visited one of those cultures in the summer of 2005 when my wife, Nicki, and I traveled with Nicole and Mike Yorkey into the Lötschental Valley, an isolated canyon high in the Alps. We spoke with the locals, many having lived in centuries-old wooden chalets with slate roofs since the day they were born. Dr. Price had studied the health patterns of the simple farmers and shepherds in the 1930s, but we weren't able to find anyone in the Lötschental Valley who remembered Dr. Price since that happened seventy-five years ago.

After analyzing these indigenous people many decades ago, Dr. Price was convinced that the standard American diet back home was sending everyone down the road to perdition. Clearly a man ahead of his time, Dr. Price posited that restoring nutrient-dense foods into our diets would do folks a world of good. When I examined Dr. Price's writings, I paid close attention to the type and form of the nutrients contained in foods—meats, dairy, fruits, vegetables, botanicals, sea vegetables, and mushrooms—that the world's healthiest people consumed.

This gave me a baseline to search for a "living" multivitamin that was the sum of nature's richest sources of these key nutrients. Although I couldn't go back to the lifestyle of our ancestors, I could certainly ingest nutrients in the forms they did and get at least part of the way there. That's why I highly recommend that you take living multivitamins in whole food form, also known as whole food or living nutrients, which are vitamins and minerals that have been fermented with probiotic microorganisms and their enzymes. (You'll find a list of such products by visiting www.BiblicalHealthInstitute.com and clicking on the GPRx Resource Guide.)

I believe everyone needs to take a living multivitamin, especially those with irritable bowel symptoms who are restricted in what foods they can eat and live with compromised digestion.

DIGESTIVE ENZYMES

Looking for a knockout blow following a one-two combination? Then consider adding digestive enzymes to your list of nutritional supplements. I always make sure I take a couple of digestive enzymes before I dig into my meals, especially when eating out. Let me explain why: When we eat raw foods, such as salad and fruit, we consume the enzymes they contain. When we eat cooked or processed meals, like in a restaurant, however, the body's pancreas must produce the enzymes necessary to digest them. The constant demand for enzymes strains the pancreas, which must kick in more enzymes to keep up with the demand. Without the proper levels of enzymes from foods—either raw or fermented—or from taking supplements, you are susceptible to excessive gas and bloating, diarrhea, constipation, heartburn, and low energy, which just happen to be some of the main symptoms of IBS.

Digestive enzymes are complex proteins involved in the digestive process. They are the body's day laborers, the ones responsible for synthesizing, delivering, and eliminating the unbelievable number of ingredients and chemicals that your body uses during the waking hours. When the body produces enzymes, their job is to stimulate chemical changes in the foods passing through the gut. The pancreas, which takes a lead role in producing digestive enzymes for the body, has to keep up by producing pancreatic enzymes.

Junk-food diets, fast chewing, and eating on the run contribute to the body's inability to produce adequate enzyme production and the subsequent malabsorption of food. These problems get worse as we age, not better. A leading biochemist, Dr. Edward Howell, cited numerous animal studies in his book *Enzyme Nutrition*, showing that animals fed diets deficient in enzymes experienced enlargement of the pancreas because the organ was working overtime to produce digestive enzymes. It wasn't long before their health was severely affected.[2]

One could eat more raw food in its natural, unprocessed state, but that isn't always possible, as I can attest when I travel or have a heavy social schedule. So if you're having trouble finding a way to eat enough raw, fresh, live foods like bananas, avocados, seeds, nuts, grapes, and other natural foods, then take plant-based digestive enzymes with each meal or snack to ease the digestion of the food. I believe digestive enzymes are essential for everyone who has digestive difficulties. (For recommended brands, visit www.BiblicalHealthInstitute.com and click on the GPRx Resource Guide.)

WHOLE FOOD FIBER

Are you taking laxatives, antacids, or antihemorrhoidal or anti-diarrhea medicines? If so, then you're a candidate for a whole food fiber supplement that supplies your body with a highly usable vegetarian source of dietary fiber. A whole food fiber supplement can counteract some of the stomach problems that cause teeth-grinding pain.

When searching for a fiber product that's right for you, choose a brand that is made from organic seeds, grains, and legumes that are fermented or sprouted for ease of digestion. One of the best ways to consume whole food fiber is to take it first thing in the morning and just before bed. Just mix it with your green superfood powder, and you've given your body more nutrition than most people get in a week. (For a list of recommended whole food fiber products, visit www.BiblicalHealthInstitute.com and click on the GPRx Resource Guide.)

GREEN FOODS

Green food concentrates, also known as green "superfoods," are supercharged concentrates of vegetables such as cereal grass juices, spinach, kale, and parsley, in addition to microalgae like chlorella and spirulina, and sea vegetables like kelp.

A combination green superfood or green food supplement is a "must have" for your daily regime. A nutritious green superfood combines the dietary benefits of whole food living nutrients and often contains whole food fiber sources, and green food powders mix well with water or your favorite fruit or vegetable juice. If you're looking for nutrition on the go before you leave the house for work in the morning, a glass of green superfood powder or a handful of caplets mixed or swallowed with water or juice provides convenient nutrition.

I'm so bullish on green foods, which do wonders for keeping you regular, that I think they should be consumed by anyone seeking digestive health.

OTHER RECOMMENDATIONS

To round out your supplements, let me propose a few more:

Omega-3 cod liver oil

One of the best sources for omega-3 fatty acids known to man, cod liver oil is an extraordinary nutritional resource that has been acknowledged to play a leading role in the development of the brain, the rods and cones of the retina of the eye, the lubrication of the joints, and the body's inflammatory response. The latter is important to digestive health.

The golden oils extracted from the filleted livers of cod and other fish, combined with wild-caught fish oils, may be an acquired taste, but after a decade of sipping spoonfuls of cod liver oil, I'm at the point where I can drink the stuff right out of the bottle. If your tender stomach can't fathom the thought of sipping omega-3 cod liver oil, you can now take this important supplement in easy-to-swallow liquid capsules. (For recommended brands, visit www.BiblicalHealthInstitute.com and click on the GPRx Resource Guide.)

Antioxidants

Antioxidants are compounds that preserve and protect other compounds in the body from free radical damage. Without going into a long explanation, free radicals are something you don't want to run rampant within your molecular system or digestive tract. Free radicals are oxygen molecules with a single electron, but these unstable molecules are known to attack the immune system's cells.

Antioxidants neutralize free radicals, which is a good thing. The most well-known antioxidants are vitamins E and C and beta-carotene. An emerging group of antioxidant rich foods and beverages, however, seems to be getting all the attention in the antioxidant category lately. Antioxidant-rich extracts from fruits such as pomegranate and beverages such as green and white tea contain plant chemicals known as polyphenols that can greatly improve health.

Herbs

Laboratory technicians peering at stool samples through microscopes usually find that one in five people have parasites. Not to send anyone screaming into the night, but I'm talking about tapeworms, pinworms, roundworms, whipworms, and hookworms. Herbs such as ginseng root, wormwood, cloves, garlics, and the green unripe hull of the black walnut are purported to rid the body of parasites.

My experience has been that people with irritable bowel syndrome can't handle these aforementioned herbs because they can upset the balance of intestinal flora in the gut. The best herbs that I've found for digestive health remain ginger, turmeric, and peppermint oil.

THE GREAT PHYSICIAN'S RX FOR IBS: SUPPLEMENT YOUR DIET WITH WHOLE FOOD NUTRITIONALS, LIVING NUTRIENTS, AND SUPERFOODS

℞

- *Consume a probiotic supplement with SBOs as part of your daily regimen.*

- *Take a whole food living multivitamin and digestive enzymes with each meal.*

- *Consume one-to-three teaspoons or three-to-nine capsules of omega-3 cod liver oil per day.*

- *Take a whole food fiber / green food blend twice per day morning and evening.*

Take Action

To learn how to incorporate the principles of supplementing your diet with whole food nutritionals, living nutrients, and superfoods into your daily life, please turn to page 72 for the Great Physician's Rx for IBS Battle Plan.

KEY #3

Practice Advanced Hygiene

When your bowels get irritable, it doesn't matter if you're about to be knighted by Queen Elizabeth—you've got to find a toilet to evacuate your large colon.

There were times when I couldn't have knelt long enough to become Sir Jordan. Having diarrhea ten, twenty, or thirty times a day overshadowed every other activity in my life. I can assure you this, however: I washed my hands after each bathroom visit, because that's what my parents had taught me ever since my days of toilet training.

Nothing is more fundamental to the human experience than using the bathroom. And when you're done, you wash your hands. Elementary, my dear Watson.

So you can imagine the emotions I felt one time when I visited the men's restroom at the Dallas-Fort Worth International Airport. After using the facilities, I approached the row of sinks to wash my hands. I was scrubbing away when I heard the stall open up behind me. I looked into the mirror and observed a burly man zip up and quickly exit the premises without washing his hands.

It's a shame that so many neglect the most fundamental rule of good hygiene, because the hands are one of the five main areas where germs enter the body—the other four being the eyes, ears, nose, and mouth. Tiny microbes find the hands and the soft tissue underneath the fingernails to be staging areas for their assault on the body's immune system. Once germs establish a beachhead on your fingertips, it's only a matter of time before you rub your eyes, scratch your nose, stroke your ears, or touch your mouth. Your body's immune system is under attack as the germs, like soldiers assaulting the beaches of Normandy, invade the portals to your body.

If you have IBS, one of the *last* things you want to do is introduce nasty squigglies that could find their way to your sensitive digestive tract. In scientific terms, this is known as auto- or self-inoculation. My suggestion is that you adopt an *advanced* hygiene system based on research done by Australian scientist Kenneth Seaton, Ph.D., who coined the phrase "Germs don't fly; they hitchhike." He believed that germs were much more likely to be spread by hand-to-hand contact as opposed to airborne exposure. To test his theory, he commenced a research study where ten healthy people were put into a room with ten other people suffering from an active virus. They spent eight hours together. There was only one caveat—no physical contact.

At the end of the day, the ten healthy people were tested, and only two were found to be infected. Dr. Seaton repeated his study with ten healthy people put into a room with ten sick people, but this time they were allowed physical contact. After eight hours, you can deduce what happened: all ten healthy people were infected after exposure through physical contact. I guess you could say that germs fly 20 percent of the time and stick out their thumbs for a ride 100 percent of the time.

Listen, you can and must take steps to protect yourself, and that starts with washing your hands properly, especially after going to the bathroom. Since I'm aware that 90 percent of germs take up residence around my fingernails, I use a creamy semisoft soap rich in essential oils.

Each morning and evening, I dip both of my hands into the tub of semisoft soap and dig my fingernails into the cream. Then I work the special cream around the tips of my fingers, cuticles, and fingernails for fifteen to thirty seconds. When I'm finished, I rinse my hands under running water, lathering them for fifteen seconds before rinsing. After my hands are clean, I take another dab of semisoft soap and wash my face. Washing my hands this way has become an everyday habit for me.

But I don't stop there because I'm aware that my face is a vulnerable entry point for germs. To combat that, I've adopted a procedure that I call a "facial dip." I fill my washbasin or a clean large bowl with warm but not hot water. When enough water is in the basin, I add one to two tablespoons of regular table salt and two eyedroppers of a mineral-based facial solution into the cloudy water. I mix everything up with my hands, then I bend over and dip my face into the cleansing matter, opening my eyes several times to allow the membranes to be cleansed. After coming up for air, I dunk my head a second time and blow bubbles through my nose. I call it "sink snorkeling."

My final two steps of advanced hygiene involve the application of very dilute drops of hydrogen peroxide and minerals into my ears for thirty to sixty seconds to cleanse the ear canal, followed by brushing my teeth with an essential oil-based tooth solution to cleanse my teeth, gums, and mouth of unhealthy germs. (For more information about my favorite advanced hygiene products, visit www.BiblicalHealthInstitute.com and click on the GPRx Resource Guide.)

℞ THE GREAT PHYSICIAN'S RX FOR IBS: PRACTICE ADVANCED HYGIENE

- *Dig your fingers into a semisoft soap with essential oils and wash your hands regularly, paying special attention to removing germs from underneath your fingernails.*

- *Cleanse your nasal passageways and the mucus membranes of the eyes daily by performing a facial dip.*

- *Cleanse the ear canals at least twice per week.*

- *Use an essential oil-based tooth solution daily to remove germs from the teeth, gums, and mouth.*

Take Action

To learn how to incorporate the principles of practicing advanced hygiene into your daily life, please turn to page 72 for the Great Physician's Rx for IBS Battle Plan.

KEY #4

Condition Your Body
with Exercise and Body Therapies

Nobody knows better than you that stress aggravates irritable bowel symptoms.

Short of selling everything you own and moving to a deserted isle in the South Pacific, what's the best stress-buster right at your fingertips?

The answer: exercise . . . good ol' heart-thumping exercise.

Now, I already know what you're thinking. *How do you expect me to go for a run when I'd have to worry about a real case of the runs? How can I even think about exercising when every time I walk I do the "clenched penguin waddle"?*

As a fellow sufferer, I will concede that there are times when a fitness workout is more unlikely than Madonna joining the Sisters of the Holy Cross. When IBS symptoms make their appearance, it's certainly easier to pack it in and veg out on the couch than pack up a duffel bag and head off to the gym. But sooner or later, when you feel up to it, you must get those arms and legs moving. Here's a short list of what exercise can do for those with IBS: (1) reduce feelings of stress; (2) improve mood through the body's release of hormones known as endorphins; (3) work the abdominal muscles, which can help the bowels return to a pattern of normal contractions; and (4) get things moving if you have constipation.

What would be the best kind of exercise? I have a background in physical fitness, having been a personal trainer at one time, so let me offer a recommendation. Unless you're young and athletic, used to pushing your body to its limits, I would steer you toward a training program called *functional fitness*, a form of gentle exercise that works your tender abdominal region, raises your heartbeat, strengthens the body's core muscles, and gives you an emotional lift at a time when life isn't so red hot.

Functional fitness can be performed within the privacy of your home, which negates any worry about having an "accident" in a gym. The idea behind functional fitness is to train movements, not muscles, through performing real-life activities in real-life positions. Functional fitness can be done with no equipment or by employing dumbbells, mini-trampolines, and stability balls. If you can feel that you can exercise outside the home, then check out functional fitness classes at gyms around the country, including LA Fitness, Bally Total Fitness, and local YMCAs. (For more information on functional fitness, visit www.GreatPhysiciansRx.com.)

Functional fitness is one of the many "body therapies" beneficial to those with IBS. There are other avenues to releasing mood-raising endorphins into your bloodstream:

Walking

Here's another gentle exercise that's tailor-made for those with IBS. Walking is especially good for those who've been lax in working out over the years. This low-impact route to fitness places a gentle strain on the hips and the rest of the body, and when it is done briskly, it makes the heart work harder and expend more energy.

If your IBS symptoms are so severe that you can ill afford being more than a few steps from the nearest toilet, then bring a treadmill into the home. That way, if you're walking up a storm only to feel a tempest brewing in your intestinal tract, you can hop off the treadmill and take care of business without having to do a lot of explaining to the friends joining you for a walk. A home treadmill also makes good sense in a frigid climate or an area where you feel unsafe walking after dark.

Rebounders

They may look like mini-trampolines, but rebounders can help you "bounce back" from IBS. Jumping on a rebounder forces you to use your abdominal muscles, and as long as your "jiggling" isn't bothering you, your stomach area will thank you for getting the blood moving. Rebounders are great for low-impact exercise and burn more calories than jogging.

Deep breathing

When you practice deep breathing, you become calmer when you breathe from your diaphragm, the muscle that separates your chest from your abdomen. I recommend sitting in a chair and concentrating on filling the lungs completely. Count to five as you breathe in; then hold your breath for several seconds before exhaling through your mouth for several more seconds.

Deep breathing relaxes your abdominal muscles, which may lead to a more normal bowel activity.

Elimination Round

When you have IBS and a bad case of the runs or stubborn constipation, you park yourself on the chamber throne a great deal. Sitting on a Western-style toilet may not be the best way to relieve your colon, however.

For centuries, people dug themselves a latrine trench or found a secluded spot behind a tree and squatted to relieve themselves. Hundreds of millions of people still "squat 'n' go" around the world today. God designed the body to squat; at the end of the rectum, there is a 90-degree bend known as the anorectal angle that is designed to prevent incontinence. When you squat, that 90-degree bend is straightened out and elimination is more complete.

Bending at the waist while sitting on a toilet is harder on your colon, however, and straining is what causes tubes of Preparation H to fly off the shelves. If you've been pushing too hard, consider using an "elimination bench" that you place in front of the toilet. When you sit on the toilet and set your feet on the foot-high bench, this places your body in a more anatomically correct squatting position.

I have an elimination bench at home and can highly recommend its use.

You Want to Sleep on It

How are you sleeping these days?

Pretty poor? I thought so.

A study by Mayo Clinic researchers found that people who have sleep disturbances are more likely to have IBS than people who don't have sleep disturbances.[1] This hardly qualifies as a surprise since IBS patients frequently complain of poor nighttime rest. It's highly disquieting to lie down in the quiet of the night and experience indigestion, abdominal stress, or frequent trips to the bathroom.

This sleep quandary is a chicken-or-the-egg thing. Do digestive ills cause insomnia or does poor sleep lead to stomach and bowel problems? Mayo Clinic researchers aren't sure, but I think they would agree with me that if you can improve the quality of your sleep, your IBS symptoms could become less . . . irritable.

How can you sleep better? Easy—go to bed earlier. If I go to bed really late, say around 2:00 a.m., I just don't feel well for a couple of days. When I get to bed before midnight, I perform better the next day. I urge you to go to bed earlier, even if it's only thirty minutes before you typically go to bed. If that means missing the local news on TV, you can catch up by reading the newspaper in the morning.

How many hours of sleep are you getting nightly? The magic number is eight hours, say the sleep experts. That's because when people are allowed to sleep as much as they would like in a controlled setting, like in a sleep laboratory, they naturally sleep eight hours in a twenty-four-hour time period.

In addition to proper sleep, the body needs a time of rest every seven days to recharge its batteries. This is accomplished by taking a break from the rat race on Saturday or Sunday. God created the earth and the heavens in six days and rested on the seventh, giving us an example and a reminder that we need to take a break from our labors. Otherwise, we're prime candidates for burnout.

LET THE SUN SHINE IN

You may not see much correlation between sunning yourself and improving your digestion, but let me explain. When your face or your arms and legs are exposed to sunlight, your skin synthesizes vitamin D from the ultraviolet rays of sunlight. The body needs vitamin D, which is not a vitamin but actually a critical hormone that helps regulate the health of more than thirty different tissues and organs, including the digestive tract. I recommend intentionally exposing yourself to at least fifteen minutes of sunlight a day to increase vitamin D levels in the body.

But if you really want to pamper yourself, then try hydrotherapy. Sitting in a sauna or taking a steam bath are forms of hydrotherapy that are beneficial, but if you're looking for an alternative approach, then consider colonic hydrotherapy to cleanse the colon and boost circulation. A therapist slowly introduces filtered water at just the right temperature into the colon, which causes accumulated toxins and impactions to release.

Hydrotherapy also comes in the form of baths, showers, washing, and wraps—using hot *and* cold water. For instance, I wake up with a hot shower in the mornings, but then I turn off the hot water and stand under the brisk, cold water for about a minute, which totally invigorates me. Cold water stimulates the body and boosts oxygen use in the cells, while hot water dilates blood vessels, which improves blood circulation and transports more oxygen to the brain. In the past, when I had major cramps around the abdomen, I would simply let a stream of hot and then cold water hit the abdominal area. I always felt better after this water massage.

Finally, pamper yourself with aromatherapy and music therapy. In aromatherapy, essential oils from plants, flowers, and spices are introduced to your skin and pores either by rubbing them in or inhaling their aromas. You can apply essential oils directly to the abdomen during an attack, which may help. The use of these essential oils will not miraculously dissipate IBS symptoms, but they will give you an emotional lift. Try rubbing a few drops of myrtle, coriander, hyssop, galbanum, or frankincense onto the palms, then cup your hands over your mouth and nose and inhale. A deep breath will invigorate the spirit.

So will listening to soft and soothing music that promotes relaxation and healing. I know what I like when it comes to music therapy: contemporary praise and worship music. No matter what works for you, you'll find that listening to uplifting "mood" music can heal the body, soul, and spirit.

℞ THE GREAT PHYSICIAN'S RX FOR IBS: CONDITION YOUR BODY WITH EXERCISE AND BODY THERAPIES

- *Make a commitment to exercise three times a week or more.*

- *Incorporate five to fifteen minutes of functional fitness into your daily schedule.*

- *Take a brisk walk and see how much better you feel at the end of the day.*

- *Make a conscious effort to practice deep-breathing exercises once a day. Inflate your lungs to full and hold for several seconds before slowly exhaling.*

- *Go to bed earlier, paying close attention to how much sleep you get before midnight. Do your best to get eight hours of sleep nightly. Remember that sleep is the most important nonnutrient you can incorporate into your health regimen.*

- *End your next shower by changing the water temperature to cool (or cold) and standing underneath the spray for one minute.*

- *Next Saturday or Sunday, take a day of rest. Dedicate the day to the Lord and do something fun and relaxing that you haven't done in a while. Make your rest day work free, errand free, and shopping free. Trust God that He'll do more with His six days than you can do with seven.*

- *During your next break from work, sit outside in a chair and face the sun. Soak up the rays for ten or fifteen minutes.*

- *Incorporate essential oils into your daily life.*

- *Play worship music in your home, in your car, or on your iPod. Focus on God's plan for your life.*

Take Action

To learn how to incorporate the principles of conditioning your body with exercise and body therapies into your daily life, please turn to page 72 for the Great Physician's Rx for IBS Battle Plan.

KEY #5

Reduce Toxins in Your Environment

Although the medical establishment has not identified the exact cause of irritable bowel syndrome, environmental and bacterial toxins in your digestive tract are among the usual suspects. Elaine Gottschall, author of *Breaking the Vicious Cycle*, wrote, "Although there is still insufficient evidence to link a specific microbe to each of the chronic intestinal disorders, it is generally agreed that intestinal microbes are not innocent bystanders."[1]

There are some mean toxins out there, just waiting for their chance to invade your gut. What kind of toxins are we talking about? You may not want to know.

In a study led by the Mount Sinai School of Medicine in New York, in collaboration with the Environmental Working Group and Commonweal, researchers at two major laboratories found an average of ninety-one industrial compounds, pollutants, and other chemicals in the blood and urine of nine volunteers.[2] A partial listing of the contaminants found in the volunteer test group revealed that many had traces of toxins such as the following:

- **PCBs.** Polychlorinated biphenyls are a group of chemical compounds developed in the 1930s for making paint, ink, dye, hydraulic fluids, and electrical transformers, to name a few uses. Despite a worldwide ban in the late 1970s, concentrations of PCBs continue

54

to be found in the fatty tissues of land animals and fish. Most farm-raised salmon are raised on pellets of ground-up fish that have absorbed PCBs from the environment.

- **Dioxins.** These organic compounds contain carbon, oxygen, and hydrogen and can be created naturally (from volcanoes and forest fires) or through the manufacturing of PVC products (plastic piping) or industrial chlorinated cleaners. This is another toxin that tends to accumulate in animals with high-fat contents such as fish and shellfish.

- **Furans.** These chemicals are country cousins to dioxins and PCBs, and although not as toxic, they are linked to problems with the endocrine (hormonal) system.

- **Metals.** Metallic particles of mercury, lead, arsenic, aluminum, and cadmium accumulate in the soft tissues of the body, which causes lowered IQs, developmental delays, and behavioral disorders. Mercury is especially prevalent in canned tuna, and arsenic can be found in tap water.

- **Asbestos.** Schools and office buildings constructed in the 1950s and '60s were insulated with this cancer-causing material. Many asbestos-infested buildings have been carefully torn down, but problems persist with the buildings still standing since the insulation in ceilings and heat ducts can crumble and release asbestos particles into the air.

- **Organochlorine insecticides.** This is a long name for pesticides such as DDT and chlordane. DDT, widely used to kill mosquitoes after World War II, was found to cause thinning of the eggshells belonging to bald eagles, peregrine falcons, and brown pelicans, resulting in deformed or broken eggs. DDT is largely banned in this country, but environmental problems have persisted for decades.

- **Phthalates.** Pronounced THA-lates, these chemicals soften plastics and lengthen the shelf life of cosmetics, hair spray, mousse, and fragrances. Phthalates harm the developing testes of males and damage the lungs, liver, and kidneys.

- **VOCs.** Volatile organic compounds, as well as semivolatile organic chemicals, are common petroleum-based chemicals present in many household products such as perfumes, aftershave lotions, toiletries, shampoos, household cleaners, furniture polishes, air fresheners, adhesives, foams, and plastics.

- **Chlorine.** Everyone who has ever swum in a municipal pool knows about chlorine, a chemical compound used as a disinfectant to kill, destroy, or control bacteria and algae. Chlorine is commonly used in municipal water supplies as well, and is found in household cleaners.

The nine volunteers in the Mount Sinai study did not work with chemicals on the job or live downwind from polluting smokestacks when they were scanned for 210 toxic substances. Of the 167 chemicals found in their blood and urine, 76 cause cancer in humans or animals, 94 are toxic to the brain and nervous system, and 79 cause birth defects or abnormal development in children. Scientists refer to this chemical residue as a person's body burden.

Although our bodies are designed to eliminate toxins, our immune systems have become overloaded to the point that they're on perpetual tilt! Presto . . . you have digestive problems. What happens is that our bodies can absorb and excrete water-soluble chemical toxins just fine, but fat-soluble chemicals such as dioxins, phthalates, and chlorine are stored in our fatty tissues, where it takes months or years for these toxins to be eliminated from our systems. This can put a massive strain on your digestive tract.

That's why the Great Physician's prescription for IBS calls for eating leaner meat since fats in meats act as chemical magnets for toxins in the environment. Certain types of fish and shellfish—including canned tuna (unless it is low mercury, high omega-3 tuna)—should be avoided to lower your exposure to mercury. Choosing organic produce will lower the level of pesticides in your body. You should thoroughly wash your fruit and veggies no matter where you do your shopping—a supermarket, health food store, or farmer's roadside stand.

Speaking of washing, nearly all municipal water is treated with chlorine, which may itself be carcinogenic and is certainly toxic because of its disinfectant ability to kill bacteria and algae. Did you know that when you take a steaming hot shower, your skin absorbs the equivalent of six to eight glasses of chlorinated water? A shower filter will protect your body from absorbing the chlorine. That's why I strongly urge the installation of shower filters with kinetic degradation fluxion (KDF) units that remove chlorine, heavy metals, and bacteria from the water. A more costly option would be installing a water filtration system in your home, which would give you filtered water every time you turn on the tap. These systems run several thousand dollars, however.

Even if you make a more modest investment of twenty dollars for a countertop water pitcher with a carbon-based filter, be sure to drink lots of water . . . *lots* of water. This will give your body the physiological ability to flush out toxins from its system. If your home is big on drinking bottled water, be aware that not all bottled waters are created equally. Some brands are nothing more than purified tap water, which means they may not be too much safer or healthier than water straight from the tap. I would shop for "spring waters" such as Mountain Valley Spring Water, Arrowhead, Deer Park, or Poland Spring, which are drawn from underground sources and thus considered more pristine.

Up in the Air

Since airborne toxins can also cause health problems, you should take steps to purify the air in your living space. Today's well-insulated homes and energy-efficient windows and doors trap "used" air with harmful particles of carbon dioxide, nitrogen dioxide, and pet dander. Opening your doors and windows to let fresh air flow into your home should be done several times a day, no matter what the temperature is like outside. Even in Florida's sticky summer heat, Nicki and I will periodically air out the house, and we'll sleep with a window cracked open in the master bedroom. We've also set up four air purifiers inside our home, which clean room air through electrical charges to capture airborne particles, microbes, and molds. Air purifiers are a wonderful technology that's becoming more affordable each year.

Carcinogenic contaminants are found in a variety of popular household products, including cleaners and cosmetics. Regarding the former, the less contact with kitchen cleansers, oven cleaner, glues, paints, paint thinner, and other solvents the better. Certain cleansers, like Ajax, along with many brands of cat litter, contain the carcinogen crystalline silica. Another popular cleanser, Comet, does not, however.

The Safe Shopper's Bible points out that household products have changed radically in the last fifty years due to scientists' ability to synthesize new chemicals from petroleum. Seventy thousand different chemical compounds are in production, and a high percentage of those accumulate in the human body, contributing to the total body burden and increasing the likelihood of cancer developing in many people.[3]

The idea is to go back to the old ways and use natural ingredients such as vinegar, lemon juice, baking soda, and commercially available natural cleansers to clean your home to a spic-and-span and high-sheen gloss. A solution of one cup of vinegar and a pail of water is all you need to mop the kitchen floor, make kitchen sinks shine, and sanitize toilets. *The Safe Shopper's Bible* is a superb resource for offering alternatives to toxin-producing products such as all-purpose cleaners, air fresheners, bathroom cleaners and disinfectants, bleaches, carpet cleaners, floor cleaners, furniture polishes, laundry detergents, and fabric softeners.

In addition, natural substitutes like lemon juice will shine up brass and copper and, when mixed with olive oil, works fine as a furniture polish. Baking soda takes on the dirty chore of scrubbing toilets, sinks, and showers as well as Mr. Clean.

Let me leave you with this thought regarding toxins in your environment. As a defense, some scientists will quote Paracelsus, the famous medieval alchemist who said hundreds of years ago, "It's the dose that makes the poison." In other words, if the toxic dose is low enough, the body can handle it.

I'm not so sure I agree with that, since I've met so many people over the years with IBS horror stories. To me, it's not a coincidence that toxins in the environment are climbing just as the ranks of those with IBS are increasing each year. That's why we must be proactive in reducing toxins in our personal environments.

℞ THE GREAT PHYSICIAN'S RX FOR IBS: REDUCE TOXINS IN YOUR ENVIRONMENT

- *Consume organically produced food as much as possible.*

- *Improve indoor air quality by opening windows, changing air filters regularly, setting out house-plants, and buying an air filtration system.*

- *Drink only purified water.*

- *Shower in purified water.*

- *Use natural products for skin care, body care, hair care, and cosmetics.*

- *Don't heat food in plastic.*

Take Action

To learn how to incorporate the principles of reducing toxins in your environment into your daily life, please turn to page 72 for the Great Physician's Rx for IBS Battle Plan.

KEY #6

Avoid Deadly Emotions

When I was a rambunctious preschooler, my mother used to put me down for a nap and play a record of the popular musical *Oliver!*, based on Charles Dickens's 1838 classic, *Oliver Twist*. The play was a touching tale of an orphan boy who runs away from a London orphanage and falls in with a gang of boy thieves run by the wizard of pickpocketry, Fagin. When the authorities catch Oliver, you wondered if the boy could be saved.

I must have listened to the soundtrack to *Oliver!* hundreds of times by the time I entered elementary school. Even years later, I can still remember the opening number sung by two dozen ragged orphans: *Food, glorious food . . . hot sausage and mustard . . . while we're in the mood . . . cold jelly and custard . . .*

I was eight years old when Mom heard that the Village Players theater group in Palm Beach, Florida, was searching for a young boy to play the role of Oliver Twist. I had never acted professionally before, but Mom was certain that I was perfect for the part. What a mob scene: we showed up at an open casting call with fifty other moms and their young sons in tow. Having listened to the musical so many times, I knew all the lines and all the songs by heart, so when it was my turn to impress the director, I was way ahead of the pack. Plus, many adults seemed to think that I had the right street urchin look.

You know the saying, "Be careful what you ask for"? Well,

after I won this key role for a major musical in South Florida, boy, was I nervous. To perform in front of all those people! We drew five hundred to eight hundred people a night for eight performances, which meant that another line from the song "Food, Glorious Food" summed things up: *Rich man have it, boys: in-di-gestion* . . . I still haven't forgotten the butterflies that fluttered around my stomach whenever the orchestra warmed up just before the rise of the curtain.

I don't recall having to run to the bathroom before an *Oliver!* performance, but it's a physiological fact that when people get nervous, they often have to have a bowel movement because the sphincter loosens its grip. There's a strong link between the emotions and gut health. "When the body's stress response kicks into high gear," says author Don Colbert, M.D., in his book *Deadly Emotions* (Thomas Nelson, 2003), "this causes the large intestine to move spontaneously, which generally results in diarrhea. Stress can also cause motility, or spontaneous movement, to decrease in the small intestines, which leads to constipation."

So there you have it: you're doomed either way by anxiety and nervousness, just two of the deadly emotions that can tie your innards up in knots. I'm not serious, of course, but I am serious about the role that emotions such as anger, acrimony, apprehension, agitation, anxiety, and alarm can play on the gut.

What about you? Are you harboring resentment in your heart, nursing a grudge into overtime, or plotting revenge against those who hurt you? If you're still bottling up emotions such as anger, bitterness, and resentment, these deadly emotions will produce toxins similar to bingeing on a dozen glazed doughnuts.

The efficiency of your immune system decreases noticeably for six hours, and staying angry and bitter about those who have teased you in the past can alter the chemistry of your body—and even prompt you to fall off the healthy food wagon again. An old proverb states it well: "What you are eating is not nearly as important as what's eating you."

This is the time to put your past in the rearview mirror and move forward. There may be someone in your past you have to forgive. I learned this lesson one time when I shared a meal with Bruce Wilkinson, the founder of Walk Thru the Bible ministries and author of *The Prayer of Jabez*. Over breakfast, he urged me to forgive those who had hurt me in the past by writing his or her name on a piece of paper and then stating, "I forgive you for . . ."

I balked at first, telling Dr. Wilkinson that I wasn't the type to hold grudges. But he persisted, asking me again, "Jordan, is there anyone in your life you need to forgive?"

Actually, there were a couple of doctors who told me that my illness was my fault. Plus, there were several relatives and friends who said they would be there for me when I got sick, but I never heard from them again. Bruce Wilkinson was right: there were more people I needed to forgive than I would have thought. So I bowed my head and asked God to help me forgive these people just as He forgives me for my sins. I prayed with a contrite heart, seeking His mercy and forgiveness.

As for you, please remember that no matter how badly you've been hurt in the past, it's still possible to forgive. "For if you forgive men their trespasses, your heavenly Father will also forgive you," Jesus said in Matthew 6. "But if you do not forgive men their trespasses, neither will your Father forgive your trespasses" (vv. 14–15).

If you're angry, hurt, or bothered by those who've been mean to you, give them your forgiveness, then let it go.

℞ THE GREAT PHYSICIAN'S RX FOR IBS: AVOID DEADLY EMOTIONS

- *Don't eat when you're sad, scared, or angry.*

- *Recognize the interaction between IBS and deadly emotions.*

- *Trust God when you face circumstances that cause you to worry or become anxious.*

- *Practice forgiveness every day and forgive those who hurt you.*

Take Action

To learn how to incorporate the principles of avoiding deadly emotions into your daily life, please turn to page 72 for the Great Physician's Rx for IBS Battle Plan.

KEY #7

Live a Life of Prayer and Purpose

If you or a loved one has been afflicted by IBS, I would imagine that you've been driven to your knees in prayer. There's something about this painful affliction—which can't be prevented and has no known medical cure—that causes one to plead for healing from the One who "fearfully and wonderfully" made us.

At times during my long struggle with a painful gut caused by Crohn's disease, my dependence upon God and prayer that He would heal me were the only things that kept me going. I believe the Lord did heal me of what one doctor called the worst case of Crohn's disease he had ever seen. I also believe that God is still in the healing business, and He listens to each and every prayer that we direct His way.

Prayer is the foundation of a healthy life, linking your mind, body, and spirit to God. Prayer is two-way communication with our Creator, the God of the universe. There's power in prayer: "The prayer offered in faith will save the sick," says James 5:15.

Start a Small Group

It's difficult to face IBS alone. If you have friends or family members struggling with similar symptoms, ask them to join you in following the Great Physician's Rx 7 Weeks of

Wellness small-group program. To learn about joining an existing group in the area or leading a small group in your church, please visit www.GreatPhysiciansRx.com.

Prayer is how we talk to God. There is no greater source of power than talking to the One who made us. Prayer is not a formality. Prayer is not about religion. Prayer is about a relationship—the hotline to heaven. We can talk to God anytime, anywhere, for any reason. He is always there to listen, and He always has our best interests at heart, because we are His children. There was something about facing my mortality that made prayer seem very real to me. When my health spun out of control and tumbled into a free fall, I didn't have much else to hang on to but the Lord. In my darkest hour, I spoke with Him constantly.

At times I felt as if I heard God's voice in reply, while on other occasions, He directed me to Scriptures that seemed particularly relevant to my dire situation. What God was teaching me was to listen to Him. Jesus said, "My sheep listen to my voice" (John 10:27 NIV), and I count myself among His flock. Another Scripture seemed particularly apt for my situation: "Blessed is the man who listens to me, watching daily at my doors, waiting at my doorway. For whoever finds me finds life and receives favor from the LORD" (Proverbs 8:34–35 NIV). Sometimes when I prayed, the Lord put things on my heart that I hadn't even thought about before I started. Sometimes He didn't answer my prayers in the way I expected Him to, but He transformed my heart to align with His.

In living a healthy, purpose-filled life, prayer is the most powerful tool that we possess. Prayer connects the entire person—body, mind, and spirit—to God. Through prayer, God takes away our guilt, shame, bitterness, and anger and gives us a brand-new start. We can eat organic whole foods, supplement our diet with whole food supplements, practice advanced hygiene, reduce toxins, and exercise, but if the spirit is not where it needs to be with God, then we will never be completely healthy. Talking to our Maker through prayer is the foundation for optimal health and makes us whole. After all, God's love and grace are our greatest foods for mind, body, and spirit.

The seventh key to unlocking your health potential is living a life of prayer and purpose. Prayer will confirm your purpose, and it will give you the perseverance to complete it. Seal all that you do with the power of prayer, and watch your life become more than you ever thought possible.

Finding His Purpose

"Living a life of purpose" is a buzz phrase these days because of a certain book you've probably read or heard about—*The Purpose-Driven Life* by Rick Warren, pastor of Saddleback Church in Lake Forest, California.

When God took me through two years of horrible sickness before restoring my health, I came out of that experience knowing what my purpose was in life: sharing God's message of health and hope so that people wouldn't have to go through what I did. Everything else that I do today is icing—made with raw honey, of course—on the cake. I can't wait to get up in the morning, hoping that I have the privilege of communicating life-changing principles of good health with one person, one thousand people, or even millions that day through television.

If you think to yourself, *I'm not sure I have a purpose,* you would be wrong. If there is breath in your lungs, you have a purpose; it's ingrained in your being. If you haven't found your purpose yet, search your heart. What makes you feel alive? What are you passionate about? The joys of family? The arts? Teaching others? Your purpose is waiting to be discovered. Pinpoint your passions, and you'll uncover your purpose. Keep in mind that God gives us different desires, dreams, and talents for a reason—we are all part of one body. Having a purpose will give you something to live for.

Don't let IBS keep you down. Many people can't say this, but I can: I know what you're going through. You can bounce back. You can overcome this affliction with God's help.

I'm cheering for you because I know you can do it. I urge you to follow the Great Physician's prescription today. I've yet to meet anyone who regretted feeling better and becoming healthier, and you won't either.

℞ THE GREAT PHYSICIAN'S RX FOR IBS: LIVE A LIFE OF PRAYER AND PURPOSE

- *Pray continually.*

- *Confess God's promises upon waking and before you retire.*

- *Find God's purpose for your life and live it.*

- *Be an agent of change in your life by adopting the 7 Keys into your life.*

Take Action

To learn how to incorporate the principles of living a life of prayer and purpose into your daily life, please turn to page 72 for the Great Physician's Rx for IBS Battle Plan.

THE GREAT PHYSICIAN'S RX FOR IBS BATTLE PLAN

DAY 1

Upon Waking

Prayer: thank God because this is the day that the Lord has made. Rejoice and be glad in it. Thank Him for the breath in your lungs and the life in your body. Ask the Lord to heal your body and use your experience to benefit the lives of others. Read Matthew 6:9–13 out loud.

Purpose: ask the Lord to give you an opportunity to add significance to someone's life today. Watch for that opportunity. Ask God to use you this day for His intended purpose.

Advanced hygiene: for hands and nails, jab fingers into semisoft soap four or five times, and lather hands with soap for fifteen seconds, rubbing soap over cuticles and rinsing under water as warm as you can stand. Take another swab of semisoft soap into your hands and wash your face. Next, fill basin or sink with water as warm as you can stand, and add one-to-three tablespoons of table salt and one-to-three eyedroppers of iodine-based mineral solution. Dunk face into water and open eyes, blinking repeatedly underwater. Keep eyes open underwater for three seconds. After cleaning your eyes, put your face back in the water, and close your mouth while blowing bubbles out of your nose. Come up from the water, then immerse your face in the water once again, gently taking water into your nostrils and expelling bubbles. Come up from the water, and blow your nose into facial tissue. To cleanse the ears, use hydrogen peroxide and mineral-based ear drops, putting two or three drops into each ear and letting stand for sixty seconds. Tilt your head to expel the drops. For the teeth, apply two or three drops of essential oil–based tooth drops to the toothbrush. This can be used to brush your teeth or added to existing toothpaste. After brushing your teeth, brush your tongue for fifteen seconds. (For recommended advanced hygiene products, visit www.BiblicalHealthInstitute.com and click on the GPRx Resource Guide.)

Reduce toxins: open your windows for one hour today. Use natural soap and natural skin and body care products (shower gel, body creams, etc.). Use natural facial care products. Use natural toothpaste. Use natural hair care products such as shampoo, conditioner, gel, mousse, and hairspray. (For recommended products, visit www. BiblicalHealthInstitute.com and click on the GPRx Resource Guide.)

Supplements: take one serving of a fiber/green superfood powder (mixed) or five caplets of a super green formula swallowed with twelve-to-sixteen ounces of water (for recommended products, visit www.BiblicalHealthInstitute.com and click on the GPRx Resource Guide).

Body therapy: get twenty minutes of direct sunlight sometime during the day, but be careful between the hours of 10:00 a.m. and 2:00 p.m.

Exercise: perform functional fitness exercises for five to fifteen minutes or spend five to fifteen minutes on a mini-trampoline. Finish with five to ten minutes of deep-breathing exercises. (One to three rounds of the exercises can be found at www.GreatPhysiciansRx.com.)

Emotional health: whenever you face a circumstance, such as your health, that causes you to worry, repeat the following: "Lord, I trust You. I cast my cares upon You, and I believe that You're going to take care of [insert your current situation] and make my health and my body strong." Confess that throughout the day whenever you think about your health condition that causes you to worry.

Breakfast

Make a smoothie in a blender with the following ingredients:

1 cup plain yogurt or kefir (goat's milk is best)

1 tablespoon organic flaxseed oil

1 tablespoon organic raw honey

1 cup organic fruit (berries, banana, peaches, pineapple, etc.)

2 tablespoons goat's milk protein powder (for recommended products, visit www.BiblicalHealthInstitute.com and click on the GPRx Resource Guide)

dash of vanilla extract (optional)

Supplements: take one capsule of a probiotic/enzyme blend with soil-based organisms and two whole food multivitamin caplets (for recommended products, visit www.BiblicalHealthInstitute.com and click on the GPRx Resource Guide).

Lunch

Before eating, drink eight ounces of water.

During lunch, drink eight ounces of water or hot tea with honey.

large green salad with mixed greens, avocado, carrots, cucumbers, celery, tomatoes, red cabbage, red peppers, red onions, and sprouts with three hard-boiled omega-3 eggs (caution: if you suffer from frequent diarrhea, too much salad is irritating to your condition, so make sure to chew very well and eliminate the cabbage, peppers, and onions)

salad dressing: extra virgin olive oil, apple cider vinegar or lemon juice, Celtic sea salt, herbs, and spices, or mix one tablespoon of extra virgin olive oil with one tablespoon of a healthy store-bought dressing

one apple with skin

Supplements: take one capsule of a probiotic/enzyme blend with soil-based organisms and two whole food multivitamin caplets.

Dinner

Before eating, drink eight ounces of water.

During dinner, drink hot tea with honey (for recommended brands, visit www.BiblicalHealthInstitute.com and click on the GPRx Resource Guide).

baked, poached, or gilled wild-caught salmon

steamed broccoli

large green salad with mixed greens, avocado, carrots, cucumbers, celery, tomato, red cabbage, red onions, red peppers, and sprouts (caution: if you suffer from frequent diarrhea, too much salad is irritating to your condition, so make sure to chew very well and eliminate the cabbage, peppers, and onions)

salad dressing: extra virgin olive oil, apple cider vinegar or lemon juice, Celtic sea salt, herbs, and spices, or mix one tablespoon of extra virgin olive oil with one tablespoon of a healthy store-bought dressing

Supplements: take one capsule of a probiotic/enzyme blend with soil-based organisms and two whole food multivitamin caplets and one-to-three teaspoons or three-to-nine capsules of a high omega-3 cod liver oil complex (for recommended products, visit www.Biblical HealthInstitute.com and click on the GPRx Resource Guide).

Snacks

apple slices with raw almond butter

one whole food nutrition bar with beta-glucans from soluble oat fiber (for recommended products, visit www.BiblicalHealthInstitute.com and click on the GPRx Resource Guide)

Drink eight-to-twelve ounces of water, or hot or iced fresh-brewed tea with honey.

Before Bed

Exercise: go for a walk outdoors or participate in a favorite sport or recreational activity.

Supplements: take one serving of a fiber/green superfood powder (mixed) or five caplets of a super green formula swallowed with twelve-to-sixteen ounces of water.

Body therapy: take a warm bath for fifteen minutes with eight drops of biblical essential oils added.

Advanced hygiene: repeat the advanced hygiene instructions from the morning of Day 1.

Emotional health: ask the Lord to bring to your mind someone you need to forgive. Take out a sheet of paper and write the person's name at the top. Try to remember each specific action that person did against you that brought you pain. Write down the following: "I forgive [insert person's name] for [insert the action he or she did against you]." After you fill up the paper, tear it up or burn it, and ask God to give you the strength to truly forgive that person.

Purpose: ask yourself these questions: "Did I live a life of purpose today?" "What did I do to add value to someone else's life today?" Commit to living a day of purpose tomorrow.

Prayer: thank God for this day, asking Him to give you a restoring night's rest and a fresh start tomorrow. Thank Him for His steadfast love that never ceases and His mercies that are new every morning. Read Romans 8:35, 37–39 out loud.

Sleep: go to bed by 10:30 p.m.

Day 2

Upon Waking

Prayer: thank God because this is the day that the Lord has made. Rejoice and be glad in it. Thank Him for the breath in your lungs and the life in your body. Ask the Lord to heal your body and use your experience to benefit the lives of others. Read Psalm 91 out loud.

Purpose: ask the Lord to give you an opportunity to add significance to someone's life today. Watch for that opportunity. Ask God to use you this day for His intended purpose.

Advanced hygiene: follow the advanced hygiene recommendations from the morning of Day 1.

Reduce toxins: follow the recommendations to reduce toxins from the morning of Day 1.

Supplements: take one serving of a fiber/green superfood powder (mixed) or five caplets of a super green formula swallowed with twelve-to-sixteen ounces of water or raw vegetable juice.

Body therapy: take a hot and cold shower. After a normal shower, alternate sixty seconds of water as hot as you can stand it, followed by sixty seconds of water as cold as you can stand it. Repeat cycle four times for a total of eight minutes, finishing with cold.

Exercise: perform functional fitness exercises for five to fifteen minutes or spend five to fifteen minutes on a minitrampoline. Finish with five to ten minutes of deep-breathing exercises. (One to three rounds of the exercises can be found at www.GreatPhysiciansRx.com.)

Emotional health: follow the emotional health recommendations from the morning of Day 1.

Breakfast

two or three eggs any style, cooked in one tablespoon of extra virgin coconut oil (for recommended products, visit www.BiblicalHealthInstitute.com and click on the GPRx Resource Guide

stir-fried onions, mushrooms, and peppers

one slice of sprouted or yeast-free whole grain bread with almond butter and honey

Supplements: take one capsule of a probiotic/enzyme blend with soil-based organisms and two whole food multivitamin caplets.

Lunch

Before eating, drink eight ounces of water.

During lunch, drink eight ounces of water or hot tea with honey.

large green salad with mixed greens, avocado, carrots, tomato, red cabbage, red onions, red peppers, and sprouts with two ounces of low mercury, high omega-3 tuna (for recommended products, visit www.BiblicalHealthInstitute.com and click on the GPRx Resource Guide) (caution: if you suffer from frequent diarrhea, too much salad is irritating to your condition, so make sure to chew very well and eliminate the cabbage, peppers, and onions)

salad dressing: extra virgin olive oil, apple cider vinegar or lemon juice, Celtic sea salt, herbs, and spices, or mix one tablespoon of extra virgin olive oil with one tablespoon of a healthy store-bought dressing

organic grapes

Supplements: take one capsule of a probiotic/enzyme blend with soil-based organisms and two whole food multivitamin caplets.

Dinner

Before eating, drink eight ounces of water.

During dinner, drink hot tea with honey.

roasted organic chicken

cooked vegetables (carrots, onions, peas, etc.)

large green salad with mixed greens, avocado, carrots, tomato, red cabbage, red onions, red peppers, and sprouts (caution: exercise caution if you suffer from frequent diarrhea)

salad dressing: extra virgin olive oil, apple cider vinegar or lemon juice, Celtic sea salt, herbs, and spices, or mix one tablespoon of extra virgin olive oil with one tablespoon of a healthy store-bought dressing

Supplements: take one capsule of a probiotic/enzyme blend with soil-based organisms and two whole food multivitamin caplets and one-to-three teaspoons or three-to-nine capsules of a high omega-3 cod liver oil complex.

Snacks

raw almonds and apple wedges

one whole food nutrition bar with beta-glucans from soluble oat fiber

Drink eight-to-twelve ounces of water, or hot or iced fresh-brewed tea with honey.

Before Bed

Exercise: go for a walk outdoors or participate in a favorite sport or recreational activity.

Supplements: take one serving of a fiber/green superfood powder (mixed) or five caplets of a super green formula (swallowed with) twelve-to-sixteen ounces of water.

Advanced hygiene: repeat the advanced hygiene instructions from the morning of Day 1.

Emotional health: repeat the emotional health recommendations from the evening of Day 1.

Purpose: ask yourself these questions: "Did I live a life of purpose today?" "What did I do to add value to someone else's life today?" Commit to living a day of purpose tomorrow.

Prayer: thank God for this day, asking Him to give you a restoring night's rest and a fresh start tomorrow. Thank Him for His steadfast love that never ceases and His mercies that are new every morning. Read 1 Corinthians 13:4–8 out loud.

Body therapy: spend ten minutes listening to soothing music before you retire.

Sleep: go to bed by 10:30 p.m.

DAY 3

Upon Waking

Prayer: thank God because this is the day that the Lord has made. Rejoice and be glad in it. Thank Him for the breath in your lungs and the life in your body. Ask the Lord to heal your body and use your experience to benefit the lives of others. Read Ephesians 6:13–18 out loud.

Purpose: ask the Lord to give you an opportunity to add significance to someone's life today. Watch for that opportunity. Ask God to use you this day for His intended purpose.

Advanced hygiene: follow the advanced hygiene recommendations from the morning of Day 1.

Reduce toxins: follow the recommendations to reduce toxins from the morning of Day 1.

Supplements: take one serving of a fiber/green superfood powder (mixed) or five caplets of a super green formula swallowed with twelve-to-sixteen ounces of water or raw vegetable juice.

Body therapy: get twenty minutes of direct sunlight sometime during the day, but be careful between the hours of 10:00 a.m. and 2:00 p.m.

Exercise: perform functional fitness exercises for five to fifteen minutes or spend five to fifteen minutes on a minitrampoline. Finish with five to ten minutes of deep-breathing exercises. (One to three rounds of the exercises can be found at www.GreatPhysiciansRx.com.)

Emotional health: follow the emotional health recommendations from the morning Day 1.

Breakfast

four-to-eight ounces of organic whole milk yogurt or cottage cheese with fruit (pineapple, peaches, or berries), honey, and a dash of vanilla extract

handful of raw almonds

one cup of hot tea with honey

Supplements: take one capsule of a probiotic/enzyme blend with soil-based organisms and two whole food multivitamin caplets.

Lunch

Before eating, drink eight ounces of water.

During lunch, drink eight ounces of water or hot tea with honey.

large green salad with mixed greens, avocado, carrots, cucumbers, celery, tomatoes, red cabbage, red peppers, red onions, and sprouts with three hard-boiled omega-3 eggs (caution: exercise caution if you suffer from frequent diarrhea)

salad dressing: extra virgin olive oil, apple cider vinegar or lemon juice, Celtic sea salt, herbs, and spices, or mix one tablespoon of extra virgin olive oil with one tablespoon of a healthy store-bought dressing

one piece of fruit in season

Supplements: take one capsule of a probiotic/enzyme blend with soil-based organisms and two whole food multivitamin caplets.

Dinner

Before eating, drink eight ounces of water.

During dinner, drink hot tea with honey.

red meat steak (beef, buffalo, or venison)

steamed broccoli

baked sweet potato with butter

large green salad with mixed greens, avocado, carrots, cucumbers, celery, tomatoes, red cabbage, red peppers, red onions, and sprouts (caution: exercise caution if you suffer from frequent diarrhea)

salad dressing: extra virgin olive oil, apple cider vinegar or lemon juice, Celtic sea salt, herbs, and spices, or mix one tablespoon of extra virgin olive oil with one tablespoon of a healthy store-bought dressing

Supplements: take one capsule of a probiotic/enzyme blend with soil-based organisms and two whole food multivitamin caplets and one-to-three teaspoons or three-to-nine capsules of a high omega-3 cod liver oil complex.

Snacks

four ounces of whole milk yogurt with fruit, honey, and a few almonds

one berry antioxidant whole food nutrition bar with beta-glucans from soluble oat fiber

Drink eight-to-twelve ounces of water, or hot or iced fresh-brewed tea with honey.

Before Bed

Exercise: go for a walk outdoors or participate in a favorite sport or recreational activity.

Supplements: take one serving of a fiber/green superfood powder (mixed) or five caplets of a super green formula swallowed with twelve-to-sixteen ounces of water.

Body therapy: take a warm bath for fifteen minutes with eight drops of biblical essential oils added.

Advanced hygiene: follow the advanced hygiene instructions from the morning of Day 1.

Emotional health: follow the forgiveness recommendations from the evening of Day 1.

Purpose: ask yourself these questions: "Did I live a life of purpose today?" "What did I do to add value to someone else's life today?" Commit to living a day of purpose tomorrow.

Prayer: thank God for this day, asking Him to give you a restoring night's rest and a fresh start tomorrow. Thank Him for His steadfast love that never ceases and His mercies that are new every morning. Read Philippians 4:4–8, 11–13, 19 out loud.

Sleep: go to bed by 10:30 p.m.

DAY 4

Upon Waking

Prayer: thank God because this is the day that the Lord has made. Rejoice and be glad in it. Thank Him for the breath in your lungs and the life in your body. Read Matthew 6:9–13 out loud.

Purpose: ask the Lord to give you an opportunity to add significance to someone's life today. Watch for that opportunity. Ask God to use you this day for His intended purpose.

Advanced hygiene: follow the advanced hygiene recommendations from the morning of Day 1.

Reduce toxins: follow the recommendations for reducing toxins from the morning of Day 1.

Supplements: take one serving of a fiber/green superfood powder (mixed) or five caplets of a super green formula swallowed with twelve-to-sixteen ounces of water.

Exercise: perform functional fitness exercises for five to fifteen minutes or spend five to fifteen minutes on a mini-trampoline. Finish with five to ten minutes of deep-breathing exercises. (One to three rounds of the exercises can be found at www.GreatPhysiciansRx.com.)

Body therapy: take a hot and cold shower. After a normal shower, alternate sixty seconds of water as hot as you can stand it, followed by sixty seconds of water as cold as you can stand it. Repeat cycle four times for a total of eight minutes, finishing with cold.

Emotional health: follow the emotional health recommendations from the morning of Day 1.

Breakfast

three soft-boiled or poached eggs

four ounces of sprouted whole grain cereal with two ounces of whole milk yogurt (for recommended products, visit www.BiblicalHealthInstitute.com and click on the GPRx Resource Guide)

one cup of hot tea with honey

Supplements: take one capsule of a probiotic/enzyme blend with soil-based organisms and two whole food multivitamin caplets.

Lunch

Before eating, drink eight ounces of water.

During lunch, drink eight ounces of water or hot tea with honey.

large green salad with mixed greens, avocado, carrots, cucumbers, celery, tomatoes, red cabbage, red peppers, red onions, and sprouts with three ounces of low mercury, high omega-3 canned tuna (caution: exercise caution if you suffer from frequent diarrhea)

salad dressing: extra virgin olive oil, apple cider vinegar or lemon juice, Celtic sea salt, herbs, and spices, or mix one tablespoon of extra virgin olive oil with one tablespoon of a healthy store-bought dressing

one bunch of grapes with seeds

Supplements: take one capsule of a probiotic/enzyme blend with soil-based organisms and two whole food multivitamin caplets.

Dinner

Before eating, drink eight ounces of water.

During dinner, drink hot tea with honey.

grilled chicken breast

steamed veggies

small portion of cooked non-gluten whole grain (quinoa, amaranth, millet, or buckwheat) cooked with one tablespoon of extra virgin coconut oil

large green salad with mixed greens, avocado, carrots, cucumbers, celery, tomatoes, red cabbage, red peppers, red onions, and sprouts (caution: exercise caution if you suffer from frequent diarrhea)

salad dressing: extra virgin olive oil, apple cider vinegar or lemon juice, Celtic sea salt, herbs, and spices, or mix one tablespoon of extra virgin olive oil with one tablespoon of a healthy store-bought dressing

Supplements: take one capsule of a probiotic/enzyme blend with soil-based organisms and two whole food multivitamin caplets and one-to-three teaspoons or three-to-nine capsules of a high omega-3 cod liver oil complex.

Snacks

apple and carrots with raw almond butter

one berry antioxidant whole food nutrition bar with beta-glucans from soluble oat fiber

Drink eight-to-twelve ounces of water, or hot or iced fresh-brewed tea with honey.

Before Bed

Drink eight-to-twelve ounces of water or hot tea with honey.

Exercise: go for a walk outdoors or participate in a favorite sport or recreational activity.

Supplements: take one serving of a fiber/green superfood powder (mixed) or five caplets of a super green formula swallowed with twelve-to-sixteen ounces of water.

Advanced hygiene: follow the advanced hygiene recommendations from the morning of Day 1.

Emotional health: follow the forgiveness recommendations from the evening of Day 1.

Purpose: ask yourself these questions: "Did I live a life of purpose today?" "What did I do to add value to someone else's life today?" Commit to living a day of purpose tomorrow.

Prayer: thank God for this day, asking Him to give you a restoring night's rest and a fresh start tomorrow. Thank Him for His steadfast love that never ceases and His mercies that are new every morning. Read Romans 8:35, 37–39 out loud.

Body therapy: spend ten minutes listening to soothing music before you retire.

Sleep: go to bed by 10:30 p.m.

DAY 5 (PARTIAL FAST DAY)

Upon Waking

Prayer: thank God because this is the day that the Lord has made. Rejoice and be glad in it. Thank Him for the breath in your lungs and the life in your body. Read Isaiah 58:6–9 out loud.

Purpose: ask the Lord to give you an opportunity to add significance to someone's life today. Watch for that opportunity. Ask God to use you this day for His intended purpose.

Advanced hygiene: follow the advanced hygiene recommendations from the morning of Day 1.

Reduce toxins: follow the recommendations for reducing toxins from the morning of Day 1.

Supplements: take one serving of a fiber/green superfood powder (mixed) or five caplets of a super green formula swallowed with twelve-to-sixteen ounces of water.

Exercise: perform functional fitness exercises for five to fifteen minutes or spend five to fifteen minutes on a mini-trampoline. Finish with five to ten minutes of deep-breathing exercises. (One to three rounds of the exercises can be foun at www.GreatPhysiciansRx.com.)

Body therapy: get twenty minutes of direct sunlight sometime during the day, but be careful between the hours of 10:00 a.m. and 2:00 p.m.

Emotional health: follow the emotional health recommendations from the morning of Day 1.

Breakfast

none (partial-fast day)

eight-to-twelve ounces of water

Supplements: take one capsule of a probiotic/enzyme blend with soil-based organisms and two whole food multivitamin caplets.

Lunch

none (partial-fast day)

Supplements: take one capsule of a probiotic/enzyme blend with soil-based organisms and two whole food multivitamin caplets.

Dinner

Before eating, drink eight ounces of water.

During dinner, drink hot tea with honey.

Chicken Soup (visit www.GreatPhysiciansRx.com for the recipe)

cultured vegetables (for recommended products, visit www.Biblical HealthInstitute.com and click on the GPRx Resource Guide)

large green salad with mixed greens, avocado, carrots, cucumbers, celery, tomatoes, red cabbage, red peppers, red onions, and sprouts (caution: exercise caution if you suffer from frequent diarrhea)

salad dressing: extra virgin olive oil, apple cider vinegar or lemon juice, Celtic sea salt, herbs, and spices, or mix one tablespoon of extra virgin olive oil with one tablespoon of a healthy store-bought dressing

Supplements: take one capsule of a probiotic/enzyme blend with soil-based organisms and two whole food multivitamin caplets and one-to-three teaspoons or three-to-nine capsules of a high omega-3 cod liver oil complex.

Snacks

none (partial-fast day)

drink eight ounces of water

Before Bed

Drink eight-to-twelve ounces of water or hot tea with honey.

Exercise: go for a walk outdoors or participate in a favorite sport or recreational activity.

Supplements: take one serving of a fiber/green superfood powder (mixed) or five caplets of a super green formula swallowed with twelve-to-sixteen ounces of water.

Advanced hygiene: follow the advanced hygiene recommendations from the morning of Day 1.

Emotional health: follow the forgiveness recommendations from the evening of Day 1.

Body therapy: take a warm bath for fifteen minutes with eight drops of biblical essential oils added.

Purpose: ask yourself these questions: "Did I live a life of purpose today?" "What did I do to add value to someone else's life today?" Commit to living a day of purpose tomorrow.

Prayer: thank God for this day, asking Him to give you a restoring night's rest and a fresh start tomorrow. Thank Him for His steadfast love that never ceases and His mercies that are new every morning. Read Isaiah 58:6–9 out loud.

Sleep: go to bed by 10:30 p.m.

Day 6 (Rest Day)

Upon Waking

Prayer: thank God because this is the day that the Lord has made. Rejoice and be glad in it. Thank Him for the breath in your lungs and the life in your body. Read Psalm 23 out loud.

Purpose: ask the Lord to give you an opportunity to add significance to someone's life today. Watch for that opportunity. Ask God to use you this day for His intended purpose.

Advanced hygiene: follow the advanced hygiene recommendations from the morning of Day 1.

Reduce toxins: follow the recommendations for reducing toxins from the morning of Day 1.

Supplements: take one serving of a fiber/green superfood powder (mixed) or five caplets of a super green formula swallowed with twelve-to-sixteen ounces of water.

Exercise: no formal exercise since it's a rest day.

Body therapies: none since it's a rest day.

Emotional health: follow the emotional health recommendations from the morning of Day 1.

Breakfast

two or three eggs cooked any style in one tablespoon of extra virgin coconut oil

one grapefruit or orange

handful of almonds

Supplements: take one capsule of a probiotic/enzyme blend with soil-based organisms and two whole food multivitamin caplets.

Lunch

Before eating, drink eight ounces of water.

During lunch, drink eight ounces of water or hot tea with honey.

large green salad with mixed greens, avocado, carrots, cucumbers, celery, tomatoes, red cabbage, red peppers, red onions, and sprouts with two ounces of low mercury, high omega-3 tuna (caution: exercise caution if you suffer from frequent diarrhea)

salad dressing: extra virgin olive oil, apple cider vinegar or lemon juice, Celtic sea salt, herbs, and spices, or mix one tablespoon of extra virgin olive oil with one tablespoon of a healthy store-bought dressing

one organic apple with the skin

Supplements: take one capsule of a probiotic/enzyme blend with soil-based organisms and two whole food multivitamin caplets.

Dinner

Before eating, drink eight ounces of water.

During dinner, drink hot tea with honey.

roasted organic chicken

cooked vegetables (carrots, onions, peas, etc.)

large green salad with mixed greens, carrots, cucumbers, celery, tomatoes, red cabbage, red peppers, red onions, and sprouts (caution: exercise caution if you suffer from frequent diarrhea)

salad dressing: extra virgin olive oil, apple cider vinegar or lemon juice, Celtic sea salt, herbs, and spices, or mix one tablespoon of extra virgin olive oil with one tablespoon of a healthy store-bought dressing

Supplements: take one capsule of a probiotic/enzyme blend with soil-based organisms and two whole food multivitamin caplets and one-to-three teaspoons or three-to-nine capsules of a high omega-3 cod liver oil complex.

Snacks

handful of raw almonds with apple wedges

one berry antioxidant whole food nutrition bar with beta-glucans from soluble oat fiber

Drink eight-to-twelve ounces of water, or hot or iced fresh-brewed tea with honey.

Before Bed

Drink eight-to-twelve ounces of water or hot tea with honey.

Exercise: go for a walk outdoors or participate in a favorite sport or recreational activity.

Supplements: take one serving of a fiber/green superfood powder (mixed) or five caplets of a super green formula swallowed with twelve-to-sixteen ounces of water.

Advanced hygiene: follow the advanced hygiene recommendations from the morning of Day 1.

Emotional health: follow the forgiveness recommendations from the evening of Day 1.

Purpose: ask yourself these questions: "Did I live a life of purpose today?" "What did I do to add value to someone else's life today?" Commit to living a day of purpose tomorrow.

Prayer: thank God for this day, asking Him to give you a restoring night's rest and a fresh start tomorrow. Thank Him for His steadfast love that never ceases and His mercies that are new every morning. Read Psalm 23 out loud.

Body therapy: spend ten minutes listening to soothing music before you retire.

Sleep: go to bed by 10:30 p.m.

DAY 7

Upon Waking

Prayer: thank God because this is the day that the Lord has made. Rejoice and be glad in it. Thank Him for the breath in your lungs and the life in your body. Read Psalm 91 out loud.

Purpose: ask the Lord to give you an opportunity to add significance to someone's life today. Watch for that opportunity. Ask God to use you this day for His intended purpose.

Advanced hygiene: follow the advanced hygiene recommendations from the morning of Day 1.

Reduce toxins: follow the recommendations for reducing toxins from the morning of Day 1.

Supplements: take one serving of a fiber/green superfood powder (mixed) or five caplets of a super green formula swallowed with twelve-to-sixteen ounces of water.

Exercise: perform functional fitness exercises for five to fifteen minutes or spend five to fifteen minutes on a minitrampoline. Finish with five to ten minutes of deep-breathing exercises. (One to three rounds of exercise can be found at www.GreatPhysiciansRx.com)

Body therapy: get twenty minutes of direct sunlight sometime during the day, but be careful between the hours of 10:00 a.m. and 2:00 p.m.

Emotional health: follow the emotional health recommendations from the morning of Day 1.

Breakfast

Make a smoothie in a blender with the following ingredients:

1 cup plain yogurt or kefir (goat's milk is best)

1 tablespoon organic flaxseed oil

1 tablespoon organic raw honey

1 cup organic fruit (berries, banana, peaches, pineapple, etc.)

2 tablespoons goat's milk protein powder

dash of vanilla extract (optional)

Supplements: take one capsule of a probiotic/enzyme blend with soil-based organisms and two whole food multivitamin caplets.

Lunch

Before eating, drink eight ounces of water.

During lunch, drink eight ounces of water or hot tea with honey.

large green salad with mixed greens, raw goat cheese, avocado, carrots, cucumbers, celery, tomatoes, red cabbage, red peppers, red onions, and sprouts with three ounces of cold, poached, or canned wild-caught salmon (caution: exercise caution if you suffer from frequent diarrhea)

salad dressing: extra virgin olive oil, apple cider vinegar or lemon juice, Celtic sea salt, herbs, and spices, or mix one tablespoon of extra virgin olive oil with one tablespoon of a healthy store-bought dressing

one piece of fruit in season

Supplements: take one capsule of a probiotic/enzyme blend with soil-based organisms and two whole food multivitamin caplets.

Dinner

Before eating, drink eight ounces of water.

During dinner, drink hot tea with honey.

baked or grilled fish of your choice

steamed broccoli

baked sweet potato with butter

large green salad with mixed greens, carrots, cucumbers, celery, tomatoes, red cabbage, red peppers, red onions, and sprouts (caution: exercise caution if you suffer from frequent diarrhea)

salad dressing: extra virgin olive oil, apple cider vinegar or lemon juice, Celtic sea salt, herbs, and spices, or mix one tablespoon of extra virgin olive oil with one tablespoon of a healthy store-bought dressing

Supplements: take one capsule of a probiotic/enzyme blend with soil-based organisms and two whole food multivitamin caplets and one-to-three teaspoons or three-to-nine capsules of a high omega-3 cod liver oil complex.

Snacks

apple slices with raw sesame butter (tahini)

one berry antioxidant whole food nutrition bar with beta-glucans from soluble oat fiber

Drink eight-to-twelve ounces of water, or hot or iced fresh-brewed tea with honey.

Before Bed

Drink eight-to-twelve ounces of water or hot tea with honey.

Exercise: go for a walk outdoors or participate in a favorite sport or recreational activity.

Supplements: take one serving of a fiber/green superfood powder (mixed) or five caplets of a super green formula swallowed with twelve-to-sixteen ounces of water.

Advanced hygiene: follow the advanced hygiene recommendations from the morning of Day 1.

Emotional health: follow the forgiveness recommendations from the evening of Day 1.

Body therapy: take a warm bath for fifteen minutes with eight drops of biblical essential oils added.

Purpose: ask yourself these questions: "Did I live a life of purpose today?" "What did I do to add value to someone else's life today?" Commit to living a day of purpose tomorrow.

Prayer: thank God for this day, asking Him to give you a restoring night's rest and a fresh start tomorrow. Thank Him for His steadfast love that never ceases and His mercies that are new every morning. Read 1 Corinthians 13:4–8 out loud.

Sleep: go to bed by 10:30 p.m.

DAY 8 AND BEYOND

If you're feeling better, you can repeat the Great Physician's Rx for IBS Battle Plan as many times as you'd like. For detailed step-by-step suggestions and meal and lifestyle plans, visit www.GreatPhysiciansRx.com and join the 40-Day Health Experience for continued good health. Or, if you want to maintain your newfound level of health, you may be interested in the Lifetime of Wellness plan. These online programs will provide you with customized daily meal-and-exercise plans and the tools to track your progress.

If you've experienced positive results from the Great Physician's Rx for IBS program, I encourage you to reach out to someone you know and recommend this book and program to them. You can learn how to lead a small group at your church or home by visiting www.GreatPhysiciansRx.com.

Remember: You don't have to be a doctor or a health expert to help transform the life of someone you care about—you just have to be willing.

Allow me to offer you this prayer of blessing paraphrased from Numbers 6:24–26:

May the Lord bless you and keep you
May the Lord make His face to shine upon you and be gracious
*   unto you*
May the Lord lift up His countenance upon you and bring you peace
In the name of Yeshua Ha Mashiach, Jesus our Messiah

Amen

Need Recipes?

For a detailed list of over two hundred healthy and delicious recipes contained in the Great Physician's Rx eating plan, please visit www.BiblicalHealthInstitute.com.

NOTES

Introduction

1. *Encyclopedia of Natural Healing*, (Burnaby, BC: Alive Publishing Group, 2002), 868.

2. Heather Van Vorous, *The First Year—IBS* (New York: Marlowe & Company, 2001).

3. "Irritable Bowel Syndrome: The Burden of Disease," from the International Foundation of Functional Gastrointestinal Disorders Web site, available at www.aboutibs.org.

4. "Survey Finds 43 Percent of Americans Suffer with Common GI Disorders," a press release from Novaris AG, released September 13, 2005, and available at http://tsedb.theglobeandmail.com/servlet/WireFeedRedirect?cf=GlobeInvestor/tsx/config&date=20050913&archive=prnews&slug=2005_09_13_11_1232_1441726.

5. "Characteristics of IBS," from the www.aboutibs.org Web site and available at www.aboutibs.org/characteristics.html.

6. Larry Trivieri Jr., ed., *Alternative Medicine: The Definitive Guide* (Berkeley, CA: Celestial Arts, 2002), 721.

7. Olafur S. Palsson, Psych. Dept. Research Associate, "Hypnosis Treatment of Irritable Bowel Syndrome," Department of Medicine, University of North California, available at www.aboutibs.org/Publications/HypnosisPalsson.html.

Key #1

1. Ron Rosedale, M.D., and Carol Colman, *The Rosedale Diet* (New York: HarperResource, 2004), 65.

2. Paul Schulick, *Ginger: Common Spice & Wonder Drug*, 3rd ed. (Prescott, AZ: Hohm Press, 1996), 36.

3. *Encyclopedia of Natural Healing* (Burnaby, BC: Alive Publishing Group, 2002), 869.

4. F. Batmanghelidj, M.D., *You're Not Sick, You're Thirsty!* (New York: Warner Books, 2003), 32.

5. Kelly James-Enger, "Sweet Stuff: How Artificial Sweeteners May Affect Your Stomach," from the msn.com Web site and available at http://acidreflux.msn.com/article.aspx?aid=64&GT1=7338.

Key #2

1. Morton Walker, "Soil-Based Organisms Support Immune System from the Ground Up," *Townsend Letter for Doctors and Patients,* August 1997.

2. Edward Howell, *Enzyme Nutrition* (Wayne, NJ: Avery Publishing, 1995).

Key #4

1. "Functional Gastrointestinal Disorders Among People with Sleep Disturbances," by the Mayo Clinic, Proc. 2004;79(12):1501-1506, and available at http://ibscrohns.about.com/gi/dynamic/offsite.htm?zi=1/XJ&sdn=ibscrohns&zu=http%3A%2F%2Fwww.mayoclinicproceedings.com%2FAbstract.asp%3FAID%3D776%26Abst%3DAbstract%26amp%3BUID%3D.

Key #5

1. Elaine Gottschall, *Breaking the Vicious Cycle* (Baltimore, ON: Krikton Press, 2004), 24.

2. "Body Burden: The Pollution in People," Environmental Working Group report, January 2003. (A complete rundown of this study, which was led by the Mount Sinai School of Medicine in New York, in collaboration with the Environmental Working Group and Commonweal, can be found at www.ewg.org/reports/bodyburden/es.php.)

3. David Steinman and Samuel S. Epstein, M.D., *The Safe Shopper's Bible* (New York: Wiley Publishing, Inc., 1995), 18.

ABOUT THE AUTHORS

Jordan Rubin has dedicated his life to transforming the health of others one life at a time. He is a certified nutritional consultant, a certified personal fitness instructor, a certified nutrition specialist, and a member of the National Academy of Sports Medicine.

Mr. Rubin is the founder and chairman of Garden of Life, Inc., a health and wellness company based in West Palm Beach, Florida, that produces whole food nutritional supplements and personal care products. He is also president and CEO of GPRx, Inc., a biblically based health and wellness company providing educational resources, small group curriculum, functional foods, nutritional supplements, and wellness services.

He and his wife, Nicki, married in 1999 and are the parents of a toddler-aged son, Joshua. They make their home in Palm Beach Gardens, Florida.

Joseph D. Brasco, M.D., has extensive knowledge and experience in gastroenterology and internal medicine. He attended medical school at Medical College of Wisconsin in Milwaukee, Wisconsin, and is board certified with the American Board of Internal Medicine. Besides writing for various medical journals, he is also the coauthor of *Restoring Your Digestive Health* with Jordan Rubin.

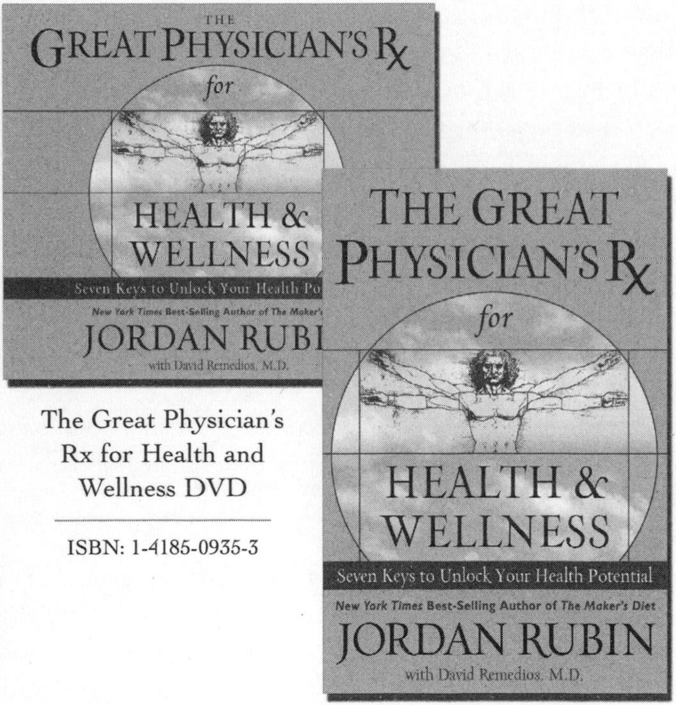

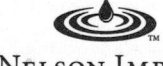

BHI

BIBLICAL HEALTH
INSTITUTE

The Biblical Health Institute (www.BiblicalHealthInstitute.com) is an online learning community housing educational resources and curricula reinforcing and expanding on Jordan Rubin's Biblical Health message.

Biblical Health Institute provides:

1. "101" level **FREE**, introductory courses corresponding to Jordan's book The Great Physician's Rx for Health and Wellness and its seven keys; Current "101" courses include:

   * "Eating to Live 101"

   * "Whole Food Nutrition Supplements 101"

   * "Advanced Hygiene 101"

   * "Exercise and Body Therapies 101"

   * "Reducing Toxins 101"

   * "Emotional Health 101"

   * "Prayer and Purpose 101"

2. **FREE** resources (healthy recipes, what to E.A.T., resource guide)

3. **FREE** media--videos and video clips of Jordan, music therapy samples, etc.--and much more!

Additionally, Biblical Health Institute also offers in-depth courses for those who want to go deeper.

Course offerings include:

   * 40-hour certificate program to become a Biblical Health Coach

   * A la carte course offerings designed for personal study and growth (launching late April 2006)

   * Home school courses developed by Christian educators, supporting home-schooled students and their parents (designed for middle school and high school ages—launching in August 2006).

For more information and updates on these and other resources go to www.BiblicalHealthInstitute.com

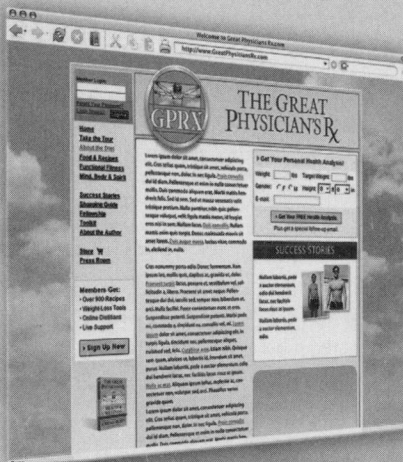
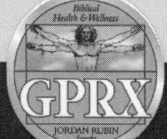

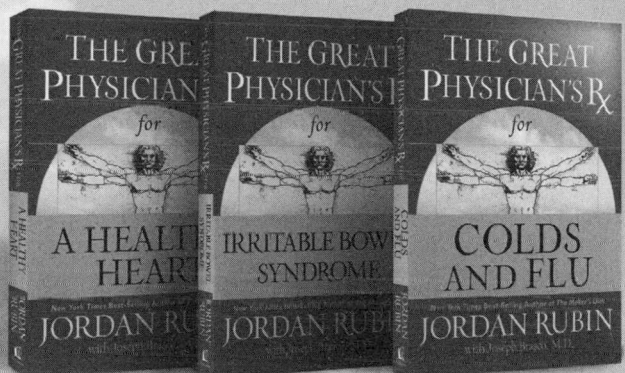
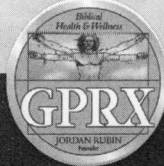

CHECK OUT THESE OTHER RESOURCES DESIGNED TO HELP YOU MAXIMIZE YOUR EXPERIENCE.

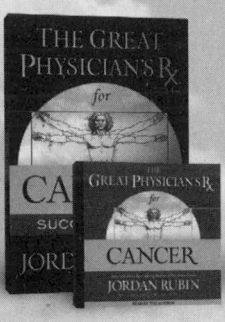 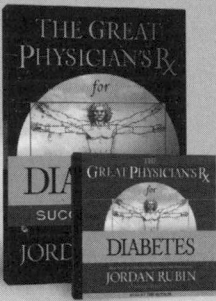 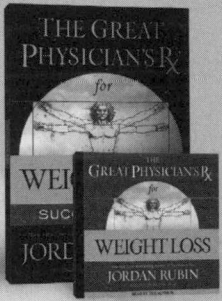

Success Guide
- Track your progress and goals
- Get helpful tips and Biblical inspiration
- Designed to help you successfully complete your experience

Audio Book
- Unabridged and read by Jordan Rubin
- Great for the car, working out or relaxing
- Makes a great gift for "non-readers"

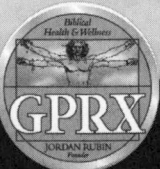

GO TO WWW.7WOW.COM
FOR ORDER DETAILS.